W9-DGI-414

Lois A. Fort Cowles, PhD

Social Work in the Health Field
A Care Perspective

"Lois Cowles has provided us with a strong review of social work's history in the health care field. Her emphasis on social work's values, Code of Ethics, and NASW standards for practice firmly root those who teach, practice, or are about to enter the social work field in today's health care system. Given today's health care and its ever-changing landscape and the pressure on social workers to perform to 'corporate' standards, this book is a refreshing reminder as well as a call to action.

Chapter 6 reflects on the practice of social work in a host institution and offers insightful comments on the needs of residents and families as well as the lone social worker practicing in a nursing home. It points to the need to provide gerontological education within the social work curriculum, as well as through continuing education for social workers working with aging populations. Cowles' perception that we also need to understand organizational priorities vs. client autonomy and be prepared to work in an interdisciplinary team are on target.

The up-to-date statistics in Chapter 8 on the status of health care insurance coverage for Americans, the autonomy, or lack thereof, for professionals, and the fragmentation of care for the insured and uninsured provide a vivid picture of the practice arena for today's social workers. The description of the 'need to create a healthier society' in Chapter 9 shows the trends we are facing as a nation.

Cowles' book reminds us of our past and the current practice of social work in health care, and 'pricks our conscience,' urging social workers to become advocates at the mezzo (community) and macro (state and national) levels for a healthier nation."

Cynthia D. Lange, MSW, CSW
Nursing home consultant
for practice and research,
Syracuse, NY

"I have found *Social Work in the Health Field: A Care Perspective* to be a well-researched presentation of this field with thorough attention paid to the knowledge, skills, values, and ethics of the social work profession and their application to our practice in the various health care settings. Lois Cowles presents these fundamentals of social work with clarity and depth as she gives the reader a thorough understanding of the historical underpinnings of social work in medicine as well as a vision of our future in this challenging area of practice.

Her conceptualization of 'caring' (rather than 'curing') and the articulation of caring social work interventions highlights our need in the profession to adapt our skills to the changing world of health care—a field requiring increasing collaboration with family caregivers, greater attention to chronic illness, and time-limited interventions necessitated by managed care.

It is my opinion that this book would give social workers interested in health care an excellent grounding for practice in this field. I would consider this a terrific text to use for graduate education—it is thorough in its coverage and current in its research and discussion of issues in the field."

Mark de St. Aubin, LCSW
Assistant Professor/Lecturer,
Graduate School of Social Work,
University of Utah,
Salt Lake City

The Haworth Press, Inc.

Social Work
in the Health Field
A Care Perspective

Social Work
in the Health Field
A Care Perspective

Lois A. Fort Cowles, PhD

The Haworth Press
New York • London • Oxford

The Haworth Press, Inc., 10 Alice Street, Binghamton, NY 13904-1580

Cover design by Dianne Hodack.

Quoted material from Kane, Robert L., Finch, Michael, Blewett, Lynn, Chen, Qing, Burns, Risa, and Moskowitz, Mark (1996). Use of post-hospital care by Medicare patients, *Journal of the American Geriatric Society,* 44(3): 242-250; reprinted with permission.

Material cited within the text from the following sources is reprinted with permission: *Health and Social Work,* copyright 1981, 1983, 1988, 1992, and 1997, National Association of Social Workers, Inc.; *NASW Clinical Indicators for Social Work and Psychosocial Services in Home Health Care,* copyright 1995, National Association of Social Workers, Inc.; *NASW Clinical Indicators for Social Work and Psychosocial Services in Nursing Homes,* copyright 1993, National Association of Social Workers, Inc.; *NASW Clinical Indicators for Social Work and Psychosocial Services in the Acute Care Medical Hospital,* copyright 1990, National Association of Social Workers, Inc.; *NASW Code of Ethics,* copyright 1996, National Association of Social Workers, Inc.; *NASW Standards for Social Work in Health Care Settings,* copyright 1987, National Association of Social Workers, Inc.; NASW Standards for Social Work Services in Long-Term Care Facilities, copyright 1981, National Association of Social Workers, Inc.

Library of Congress Cataloging-in-Publication Data

Cowles, Lois A. Fort.
   Social work in the health field : a care perspective / Lois A. Fort Cowles.
     p. cm.
   Includes bibliographical references and index.
   ISBN 0-7890-6033-7 (hardcover : alk. paper) — 0-7890-0913-7 (pbk. : alk. paper)
   1. Medical social work. I. Title.
HV687.C68 1999
362.1'0425—dc21
                                            99-16078
                                            CIP

CONTENTS

Chapter 1

Orientation to Social Work in the Health Field

HISTORICAL BACKGROUND AND DEVELOPMENT

The Birth of Social Work in Health Care

Social work in health care began in the hospital setting in 1905 when a nurse, Garnet I. Pelton, was appointed by a physician, Richard C. Cabot, to fill the first hospital social worker position at Massachusetts General Hospital (MGH) in the Internal Medicine Clinic (Cannon, 1923, cited in Cowles, 1990:2). Two years later, in 1907, social work services were placed in the Neurology Clinic of MGH, and this event is sometimes heralded as the beginning of social work in mental health (Stuart, 1997:26). However, there is little evidence that anyone at the time made a distinction between medical and psychiatric social work.

According to Ida Cannon (1923), who soon succeeded Garnet Pelton in the social worker position and became a pioneer in hospital social work, the birth of social work in hospitals was closely related to the extension of medical practice from the physician's office and home visits to the hospital as the setting for medical diagnosis and treatment. An effect of this change, which occurred around the turn of the century, was what Cannon called "a constriction of the field of vision" of the physician (1923:30). The physician was cut off from observation of patients in the context of their homes, work, and other life situations. Thus, the physician was left to focus primarily on physical factors (Cowles, 1990).

Social work in hospitals was conceptualized as a means of compensating for this deficit by having its practitioners bring pictures of patients as people in their customary settings to the awareness of the medical and nursing staff. According to Cannon (1923:14), Dr. Cabot saw the potential for social work in hospitals to be "a potent means for more accurate diagnosis and more effective treatment" (cited in Cowles, 1990:3). Cannon described this function of hospital social work as follows:

> It seeks to understand and to treat the social complications of disease by establishing a close relationship between the medi-cal care of patients in hospitals or dispensaries and the services of those skilled in the profession of social work, [in order] to bring to the institutionalized care of the sick such personal knowledge of their social condition as will hasten and safe-guard their recovery. (1923:i)

In a speech titled "Hospital and Dispensary Social Work" deliv-ered at the International Conference of Social Work held in Paris, France in July 1928, Dr. Cabot agreed that a primary function of hospital social work was teaching doctors and nurses about "the social and psychological aspects of disease" (Cabot, 1928:265).

Early Seeds of Role Conflict

However, the seeds for a disagreement that lingers today between physicians and social workers concerning the hospital social worker role are evident when other expectations of Cannon (1923) and Cabot (1928) are compared.

The difference was that Cannon expected the social worker role to include the direct treatment of the patient's social and psycholog-ical problems which were among the causes or effects of their health problems or which acted as barriers to cooperation with the medical treatment plan:

> the social worker seeks to remove those obstacles in the pa-tient's surroundings, or in his mental attitude, that interfere with successful treatment, thus freeing him to aid in his own recovery. (1923:15)

This view of the social worker's role is evident also in Cannon's reference to

> the need for the cooperation of one skilled in understanding social problems, and equipped by training and experience to guide a patient in solving those personal ones, that may arise from his illness or to which his illness may have been due in part . . . (1923:30)

In contrast, when Cabot spoke of the main functions of hospital social work, he described the social worker as a liaison or bridge between the hospital and the social environment and community resources of the patient:

> For one of the chief functions of such a department [hospital social work] is to connect the hospital with all the social forces and helpful agencies outside its walls. (1928:260)

Similarly, Cabot expected the hospital social worker to help patients adjust to hospitalization (e.g., to explain the hospital system to patients and provide reassurance if they were frightened by it, and to explain their health condition to them if it appeared the medical and nursing staff had not adequately done so) and to help patients adjust to returning home (e.g., help patients and their families understand the implications of the patients' health condition for the posthospital stage, such as the expected length of disability) (1928:262-263).

In short, Cabot (1928) expected the role of the social worker to revolve around "bridging the gap" between the hospital environment and the usual social environment of the patients in order to remove barriers to effective medical treatment, while Cannon (1923) additionally expected the hospital social worker role to include efforts to modify any social environmental or emotional causes or effects of the patients' health condition.

Growth of Social Work in Health Care

In Hospitals

From this beginning with one social worker in one hospital in 1905, social work had emerged in 100 hospitals by 1913 and in 400 by 1923 (Cannon, 1923:vii). By 1994, 77 percent of psychiatric hospitals and 88 percent of general acute-care hospitals reported having social work services (American Hospital Association, 1997). Although the majority of all types of hospitals claim to have social work services, the 1995 National Association of Social Workers (NASW) membership survey results indicate that only 18.2 percent of respondents name their primary practice setting as nonpsychiatric inpatient facilities and less than 1 percent (0.7 percent) report their primary practice setting as an inpatient mental health facility (Gibelman and Schervish, 1996:94).

Overall Practice Settings and Practice Areas

An earlier membership survey by the NASW in 1982 found that mental health was the largest practice area of its then approximately 90,000 members (26.6 percent), while the physical health field was second largest (18.1 percent) indicating that nearly 45 percent (44.7 percent) of NASW members were practicing in mental or physical health care (Gibelman and Schervish, 1996:94).

Data from the 1995 NASW membership survey indicated that mental health continues to be identified by social workers as the largest social work *practice area*, with 39 percent so naming it, and another 12.9 percent named medical health as their primary practice area (coming in third after "family and children's services"—24.9 percent of NASW members responding), indicating that 51.9 percent of NASW members most recently report their primary practice area as mental or physical health care (Gibelman and Schervish, 1996:94).

However, it should be pointed out that less than 4 percent (3.2 percent) of all 1995 survey respondents classified their primary *practice setting* as either inpatient or outpatient mental health, while a total of 34.6 percent classified their primary practice setting as a medical health one. Inpatient medical facilities (hospitals) were named by 18.2 percent of respondents as their primary practice setting, second only to "social services agencies," named by 20.5 percent (Gibelman and Schervish, 1996:94).

This suggests some discrepancy between what social workers consider their "practice area" and their "practice setting." Perhaps an increasing percentage of clinical social workers in health care settings have come to think of themselves as practicing in mental health more than "health care." In addition, many clinical social workers in private social work practice probably classify their practice area as mental health.

The First Specialty Area and Secondary Setting of Social Work

Social work in the health field has the distinction of being the first specialty area of social work practice, which also marked the entry of social work into *secondary settings* of practice, or settings in which the primary organizational function is not social work but another function, such as medical care, education, law enforcement, or business and industry.

In 1918, hospital social workers banded together to form the American Association of Hospital Social Workers (AAHSW), which published the journal *Hospital Social Service* from 1919 until 1933 (Bracht, 1978:11, 14). In 1955, the AAHSW merged with other specialty groups and with the American Association of Social Workers (AASW) to become the National Association of Social Workers (NASW) (Popple and Leighninger, 1993:72).

Currently, two specialty journals of social work in health care are published: *Health and Social Work*, a publication of the NASW, and *Social Work in Health Care*, published by The Haworth Press. On their inside front covers, both journals broadly define health care to include both mental and physical health care. Currently, the major national specialty organization in health care is the Society for Social Work Leadership in Health Care, formerly known as the Society for Social Work Administrators in Health Care (SSWAHC) of the American Hospital Association, founded in 1965.

The Separation of Medical from Psychiatric Social Work

What little literature exists concerning the development of psychiatric social work suggests that prior to the 1920s, social workers employed in medical and psychiatric clinics were engaged in much the same type of role and function as described earlier by Cannon (1923) and Cabot (1928), that is, providing relevant social environmental information concerning patients to nurses and physicians, facilitating patient discharge and posthospital adjustment, and linking patients and families with needed community resources. This is reflected in the following commentary on early psychiatric social work:

> Before 1920 psychiatric social work was based on the assumption that a knowledge of the social environment was vital to an understanding of individual behavior. The gathering of such information by means of social casework was, in theory, the primary function of the specialty. In practice, however, social casework was fluid rather than fixed. The daily activities of social workers centered on providing assistance and aid to distressed individuals and to help them take advantage of a variety of supportive services. (Grob, 1983:250)

What began as "social work in health care" eventually divided into medical and psychiatric social work, a division stimulated by the introduction of Freudian psychoanalytic concepts around 1920. This division was further solidified by the acceleration of the mental hygiene movement following World War I, which involved the rapid expansion of psychiatric hospital and home services to returning servicemen (Lubove, 1965:76, 89). Many servicemen were suffering from what was then called "shell shock," but is now labeled post-traumatic stress syndrome.

Freudian theory began to be popular in America around 1920, at a time when social workers were in the throes of distress over Abraham Flexnor's 1915 address to them. Flexnor asserted that social work was not a "profession" because it did not have a body of knowledge rooted in science and did not focus on direct services to individuals, as much as on environmental modification and consultation and linkage of clients to other direct-service providers (Trattner, 1989:234-235). Flexnor's message stimulated a struggle within the social work profession to make the needed changes to win professional status. It also marked a beginning rift between practitioners who continued to see the basic mission of social work as improving environmental conditions for people and those who sought professional status through shifting to a focus on person-centered problems, with a psychoanalytic theory base.

A training school for psychiatric social work was established at Smith College in 1918 (Lubove, 1965:78), and in 1922, a section on psychiatric social work was organized within the American Association of Hospital Social Workers (Lubove, 1965:127).

Following both World War I and World War II, thousands of servicemen returned home to the United States with psychological injuries as well as physical ones. Veterans Administration (VA) hospitals rapidly expanded after World War II, and large numbers of social workers were employed by them, as both medical and psychiatric social workers.

Then, *the deinstitutionalization movement,* a push to reduce the population of mental institutions and to transfer the patients to community-based care, took off in the 1950s. A variety of events combined to provide the momentum for change, including the growing recognition that (1) America's mental hospitals were overcrowded, (2) they were more warehouses than treatment or rehabilitation centers, (3) their bureaucratic organization tended to add *secondary* disabilities (i.e., those resulting from social responses to people with primary disabilities) to the primary mental dysfunction, and (4) their cost to the taxpayers had reached alarming proportions. The movement culminated in the *serendipitous* (i.e., a happy accident) discovery of *psychotropic drugs* (i.e., drugs that alter mood or mental functioning), which made it possible to consider community-based treatment as an alternative to institutionalization (Trattner, 1989:187-188).

The Community Mental Health Center (CMHC) Program accompanied the deinstitutionalization movement. The program began with the passage of the Community Mental Health Services Acts of 1963 and 1965, which provided for the nationwide development of federal and state tax-funded, community-based, comprehensive mental health service centers (Karger and Stoesz, 1998:340-341).

This development of community mental health centers, similar to the earlier expansion of VA hospitals, provided greatly increased job opportunities in social work, especially in "psychiatric" social work. Unfortunately, however, during the Reagan administration of the 1980s, the federal government share of CMHC funding dropped from 24 percent in 1976 to 2 percent by 1984. Many states were unable to make up the difference, and as a result, the original intent of the centers to provide comprehensive services to everyone who needed them, with an emphasis on prevention and early intervention, had to be downsized to publicly funded services only for the most seriously disturbed (Karger and Stoesz, 1994:321).

Since its inception in 1905 in the general hospital setting, social work in the health field has expanded to include practice in a variety of health care settings, such as psychiatric and other specialty hospitals, public health agencies, nursing homes and rehabilitation centers, health maintenance organizations, community-based clinics, private medical practice, home care agencies, and hospice programs. Whereas in 1983 about 75 percent of medical social workers were employed in hospitals (NASW, 1983), and the majority of psychiatric social workers (i.e., clinical social workers) were presumably employed in community mental health centers, by 1992, the U.S. Department of Labor reported 474,176 employed social workers in the United States, of which 26.02 percent, or 123,372, were in health services. The employment distribution across health care settings is shown in Table 1.1.

The data in Table 1.1 show that by 1992, only about 54.3 percent of health care social workers were employed in hospitals, probably reflecting the downsizing of acute inpatient hospital care as part of the nation's cost-containment efforts.

THEORETICAL PERSPECTIVES

The Person-in-Environment Perspective

The unifying theoretical perspective at the root of all current social work practice is the view that people can best be understood and helped in the context of the conditions and resources of their social environment.

Social environment refers to the quality and characteristics of one's life situation, including interpersonal relationships, resources for one's needs, and one's positions, roles, and participation in the society. More specifically, the social environment encompasses things such as family and home life, employment and income, school situation and educational opportunities, housing and utilities, social welfare resources in the community, opportunities for political participation, access to health services, relationships with neighbors and friends, police protection and crime control, and recreational resources.

TABLE 1.1. Practice Settings of Health Care Social Workers, 1992

Types of Practice Settings	Percent of all social workers in various health settings	Number of health care social workers in each setting	Percent of health care social workers in each setting
Physician's office	1.48	7,025	6.0
Other health professional's office	1.22	5,805	5.0
Nursing/personal care facility	2.99	14,200	12.0
Hospital, public or private	14.13	67,022	54.3
Medical or dental laboratory	0.01	51	0.04
Home health care service	0.90	4,257	4.0
Allied health service	5.28	25,013	20.0
TOTAL	26.02	123,372	100.0

Source: Ginsberg, Leon (1995). *The Social Work Almanac* (Second Edition). Washington, DC: NASW Press, 355. Data obtained from U.S. Department of Labor, Bureau of Labor Statistics, November 1993.

Sociologists speak of social institutions or social systems when they refer to the economy, politics, the family, education, health care, transportation, and religion. These are abstractions that characterize the mechanisms through which society provides for its members' basic needs. In a sense, describing a person's social environment means describing his or her situation in life relative to the social institutions of the society.

In "real life," the nature of these social institutions is *manifest* (revealed) in business and industry, employment opportunities, wage levels, schools, police departments, courts and correctional facilities, religious organizations, health service facilities, a variety of housing types and conditions, and families with a range of cultures, structure, composition, and level of functioning. It is these "real-life manifestations" to which social workers refer when speaking of the social environment.

Social workers believe that individuals, including their attitudes, feelings, values, beliefs, behaviors, mental and physical health status, and their functioning in social roles in their families, work-places, schools, neighborhoods, and so forth, can best be understood by taking into account their social environmental situation, as described in the previous paragraph. This belief is called the *person-in-environment perspective.*

The Biopsychosocial Model and the Medical Model

Beginning with the work of Ida Cannon at the Massachusetts General Hospital in the early 1900s, the underlying theoretical perspective of social work in the health field has been that physical, psychological, and social environmental conditions tend to influence one another and must be taken into account in order to understand and help clients and their families in health settings. This is called the *biopsychosocial model.*

The biopsychosocial perspective is similar to the person-in-environment perspective. The person-in-environment concept claims that people both affect and reflect their social environment, and this depicts the *dual focus* of the social work profession. The biopsychosocial perspective is an elaboration of the person-in-environment view; it suggests that a "person" has both psychological and physical components that combine to interact with the social environment.

The biopsychosocial perspective is sometimes referred to as a *holistic* view because it seeks to encompass the "whole picture" of a person. It is often contrasted with the so-called *medical model* that focuses on physical aspects of health problems. Another difference between the medical and biopsychosocial models is that the medical model is focused on physical or mental "disease" in the individual, while the biopsychosocial model is also attuned to the social environmental causes and effects of health problems.

The biopsychosocial model also is an example of *general systems theory* because it views a person's health status as reflecting the interdependency of physical, psychological, and social environmental systems. General systems theory holds that all levels of organization in nature are linked so that change in one affects change in the others (Engel, 1977).

Social workers in health care settings are concerned with the interaction of physical, psychological, and social conditions of the client, both as causes and effects. A social situation or life change event (such as marital dysfunction, social isolation, loss of one's job, or death of a loved one) can produce emotional distress that can lead to changes in physical functioning that increase one's vulnerability to disease. On the other hand, a physical health problem can erode self-confidence or interfere with the ability to perform customary activities, which can affect work, marriage, or other social roles and relationships and, in turn, lead to emotional distress.

Health Care and Medical Care

The distinctions between the biopsychosocial model and the medical model are related to the distinction between *health care* and *medical care*. A common failure to understand this difference is one of the problems in the U.S. health care system.

Medical care is what physicians provide in the course of monitoring patient health and diagnosing and treating health problems. *Health care* refers to individual and societal efforts to prevent health problems from emerging and to maintain current levels of health. Examples include individuals' efforts at proper diet and exercise, weight control, adequate rest and relaxation, safety precautions, and avoidance of intake of hazardous chemicals. In addition, health care requires provision of an environment that is supportive of physical needs, personal development, and social integration, as well as free of environmental pollution in all its forms.

In other words, "health care" requires both personal responsibility to choose a healthy lifestyle and social provision of the necessary resources and conditions to enable successful individual efforts. The World Health Organization (WHO) has taken the position that "health is a state of complete physical, mental, and social well-being and not merely the absence of disease or infirmity" (World Health Organization, 1978).

Curing and Caring

Much of medical care is repair work for existing health problems. Unfortunately, few serious health problems can be cured (McLachlan and McKeown, 1971:48). Today, the major health problems are chronic rather than acute infectious diseases, as in the early 1900s when social work in health care began.

Essentially, *curing and caring* are the two basic approaches to helping with health and other human problems. Curing refers to efforts to correct the underlying condition. Caring refers to the provision of supportive assistance to (1) promote healthy growth and development, (2) sustain function and relieve distress during a temporary problem episode, and (3) maximize comfort and function when a problem is permanent or even terminal. Although caring is not limited to any particular level of health service, medical care is primarily focused on the secondary level of repair of acute problems (see Chapter 4).

Levels of Health Service and Associated Practice Settings

The health care delivery system has three basic levels of services that represent stages of health status: primary, secondary, and tertiary. These stages revolve around (1) prevention, (2) repair, and (3) compensation.

Primary care, the first level of health service, is focused on primary prevention and health maintenance, that is, preventing health problems from emerging and providing very early intervention. Associated practice settings for social workers and other health professionals include public health agencies, private medical practice (general practice, family practice, internal medicine, and pediatrics), outpatient clinics, and health maintenance organizations (HMOs).

Secondary care, the second level of health service, is focused on secondary prevention, or preventing health problems that have already emerged from developing into a worsened state, that is, repair and control. Hospitals and other residential treatment centers are the main settings of secondary care.

Tertiary care, the third and last level of health service, is focused on providing supportive assistance to maximize the comfort and function of persons with well-advanced health problems that cannot be cured, being either chronic or terminal in nature. The practice settings associated with tertiary care include rehabilitation centers, nursing homes, hospice programs, home care agencies, and day care centers.

However, in recent years, it has become less clear which settings are associated with which levels of health service. Hospital emergency rooms and outpatient clinics have increasingly become centers of "primary care," especially for the poor. In addition, both nursing homes and home care agencies have begun to serve an increasing number of persons whose conditions are neither chronic nor terminal, but who are merely recovering from an acute episode of a health problem, such as after an injury or surgical procedure.

HUMAN DIVERSITY AND BEHAVIOR

Human diversity refers to the fact that people vary, one from another, on a multitude of biopsychosocial dimensions, such as age, gender, racial identity, ethnicity or culture, sexual orientation, religious beliefs and practices, and socioeconomic class (assessed by education, occupation, and income). People also vary in intelligence, talents, interests and hobbies, physical appearance and size, genetic make-up, physical and mental health status, personality traits and coping mechanisms, personal norms and values, support groups and reference groups, rural or urban background, family structure and composition, and relationships, as well as history of life events and experience. *Sensitivity to human diversity* means being knowledgeable about, attentive to, and respectful of differences in culture, perception, and behavioral patterns that may be associated with human variation and individualizing every person (i.e., in working with them, take into account all that makes them special).

It is important in all social work practice to be sensitive to human diversity variables because, otherwise, we cannot truly understand people or their behavior, nor can we work with them effectively. Sensitivity to human diversity is important in health care settings because these variables play important roles in (1) health behavior, (2) illness behavior, and (3) sick-role behavior.

Health behavior refers to what a person does, or does not do, in an effort to take care of his or her health. Illness behavior involves how a person interprets and responds to signs and symptoms of health problems. Sick-role behavior is a person's behavior following determination of illness or injury.

Relevance of Human Diversity Variables and Behaviors to Social Work Practice

Social workers who practice in health service settings provide a variety of direct services to patients and their families, which will be discussed in Chapter 2. In the course of providing these direct services, it sometimes becomes evident that the patient or family is engaging in behaviors that (1) seem to endanger the patient's health, (2) suggest a lack of attention or excessive attention to "symptoms" or represent unconventional methods of treatment, or (3) indicate lack of compliance with medical recommendations as to, for example, diet, activity, medications, and "stress."

Health behavior can be influenced by such variables as income, education, ethnicity, religion, occupation, intelligence, age, and sexual orientation. Illness behavior can reflect a person's gender, age, mental health status, or ethnicity. Whether a person seeks help from a neighbor, physician, chiropractor, midwife, or spiritual healer can be influenced by social class, religious beliefs, ethnicity, or rural/urban location. Finally, sick-role behavior, such as whether a person's behavior complies with medical or other health service provider recommendations, can be affected by such variables as social class, religious beliefs, ethnicity, available social supports, and gender.

In mental health care settings, where social workers are among the primary providers of health treatment services, such behaviors are an integral concern. In physical health care settings, health behavior, illness behavior, and sick-role behavior are primarily the concern of the medical and nursing staff. However, medical social workers may become involved with these behaviors while assisting patients and their families with such social work services as (1) preadmission planning, (2) discharge planning, (3) adjustment to the health care setting or service, (4) adjustment to the diagnosis, prognosis, or medical treatment plan, or (5) helping them to understand and make decisions concerning treatment-related issues.

It is helpful for social workers to be familiar with the literature concerning human diversity as it relates to general differences in human behavior. However, workers must take care not to assume that because a person is of a particular racial or ethnic group, religion, gender, age, social class, and so on, that he or she necessarily believes in certain things, adheres to certain customs, or behaves in a prescribed manner. Every human being is a multifaceted individual.

INTERDISCIPLINARY TEAMWORK

Multidisciplinary Organizations

All health service settings are *multidisciplinary*, except perhaps private practice involving one discipline of one professional group. A *multidisciplinary* setting means that more than one professional group or more than one *discipline* (specialty) within a professional group are working in the same setting.

The Interdisciplinary Concept

However, multidisciplinary settings are not necessarily *interdisciplinary*; interdisciplinary means that various professions or disciplines are working together and collaborating rather than merely working in the same place.

Models of Collaboration

Interdisciplinary teamwork is the "consensus" form of *collaboration* (co-laboring or working together). Mailick and Jordon (1977) refer to three models of collaboration: (1) *the authoritarian model* (e.g., an operating-room team); (2) *the matrix model* (casual, informal, low-contact interaction among any number of professionals), and (3) *the consensus model* (interdisciplinary teamwork, which relies heavily on joint decision making).

Characteristics of Interdisciplinary Teamwork

Theoretically, interdisciplinary teamwork is distinguished from other forms of collaboration by (1) small group size, (2) the operation of small-group dynamics (such as a sense of group bond), (3) shared decision making, and (4) more frequent, regular, and direct face-to-face communication (Mailick and Jordon, 1977).

Interdisciplinary Teams As a Form of Group Practice

Interdisciplinary teamwork is a form of group practice (Rubin and Beckhard, 1972). It revolves around services to a particular patient or client and does not include routine staff meetings (which usually concern staff "business"). Interdisciplinary teamwork is an alternative to one person of one professional group trying to be "all things" to the patient; it also is an alternative to several persons being involved without planning and intervening in a collaborative manner.

Social workers in health care settings often are asked to serve on interdisciplinary teams, and sometimes to lead them (Kane, 1978, 1980). The core of such teams usually consists of all, or representatives of, the professional staff who are working with the same patient or whose expertise is considered relevant. In addition, such teams may include some of the nonprofessional staff who are providing "hands-on" care to the patient as well as the patient and some family members.

Background of Interdisciplinary Teamwork in Health Settings

Interdisciplinary health care teams first emerged in community mental health centers and expanded to general hospitals, rehabilitation centers, nursing homes, and other health service settings (Harris, Saunders, and Zasorin-Conners, 1978).

Several developments in the field of health care combined to promote the concept of interdisciplinary teamwork. One of these was the increased specialization and division of labor (Nagi, 1978). Where once there were only general practitioners, multiple medical and surgical specialties grew. Where once hospitals were staffed mostly by physicians and nurses, a variety of other professions, paraprofessions, and technician types of occupations emerged. This increased specialization and division of labor resulted in one patient sometimes having several physicians and other kinds of personnel involved in his or her care.

A second development that contributed to the idea of health care teams was the expanding scope of the concept of "health" (Nagi, 1978), from thinking of it as the absence of physical disease to include a healthy environment and lifestyle, weight control, adequate exercise, satisfactory social-role functioning, a positive mental outlook, satisfying involvement in personal development, and a general sense of well-being.

A third factor was the growing recognition that human problems tend to be *complex* (multiple) rather than *simple* (singular). As a purely hypothetical example, a patient whose main problem seems to be a diseased gall bladder that requires surgical removal may also have a chronic obesity problem, a tendency to eat too much fat, a lack of regular exercise, be socially isolated, and have marriage problems. Or, a person who is diagnosed as having schizophrenia may also be alcoholic, homeless, malnourished, have a venereal disease, be estranged from family or friends, and without income, support, or occupation.

Finally, a fourth recognition that led to interdisciplinary teamwork, which is related to the third, is that such clusters of problems often are interdependent and constitute a "pathology system," so that one cannot effectively treat one problem without addressing them all (Nagi, 1978; Platt, 1994).

As Platt has noted:

> In health, the nature of problems related to the so-called new morbidity—chronic disease, emotional problems, recurrent illness—and an appreciation of the interaction among social, emotional, and biologic factors require both a new framework for problem analysis and a new way of practice. Systems theory provides the framework for analysis, and a team approach provides a method for practice. (1994:5)

To paraphrase Briggs (1997:19), the effective interdisciplinary health team, as with all effective small groups, is "synergistic" in the sense that *the potential power and product of each member is enhanced by its interaction and cooperation with that of the other members.*

Rationale for Interdisciplinary Teamwork

The rationale for interdisciplinary teamwork is that multiple kinds of knowledge and skill need to be involved and coordinated to maximize efficiency and effectiveness (Jonas, 1981). *Efficiency* refers to "getting the most for the buck," that is, the least waste and cost, relative to the outcome or benefit. On the other hand, *effectiveness* involves a successful outcome in terms of what one aimed to achieve. Thus, the efficiency and/or effectiveness *objectives of interdisciplinary teamwork* include comprehensive and coordinated service delivery, optimal use of manpower, improved quality of patient care, "whole person" care, and cost savings by reducing gaps and overlap in services (Friedson, 1978). As a result, "The recipient of services, the team member, the profession, and society as a whole all benefit from interprofessional collaboration" (Julia and Thompson, 1994b:53).

Functions of Interdisciplinary Teams

The functions of such teams include (1) shared assessment of patient problems and needs, (2) exchange of relevant information, (3) team teaching of clients/patients, (4) ethical decision making, (5) development of intervention plans, (6) delegation of tasks and responsibilities, (7) modification of plans as needed, and (8) evaluation of outcome (Bope and Jost, 1994).

Common Problems in Interdisciplinary Team Functioning

Interdisciplinary teams may encounter at least six problems: (1) turf protection, (2) different values and perceptions of the problems and needs, (3) self-promotion, (4) prestige and status discrepancies that impair open communication, (5) lack of understanding of one another's language, skills, and knowledge areas, and (6) differences in the problem-solving process (Julia and Thompson, 1994a).

Teamwork Requirements

Finally, in order for interdisciplinary teams to work well, a number of requirements, which have been identified in a variety of sources (Given and Simmons, 1977; Kane, 1978; French, 1979; Rubin and Beckhard, 1972; Sheps, 1974; Julia and Thompson, 1994b; Briggs, 1997), should be met, including the following:

1. Role clarity, but role flexibility
2. Mutual respect and trust
3. Consensus on group norms, values, commitment, and purpose
4. An egalitarian attitude; a sense of equal importance
5. A sense of group bond and interdependence, not autonomy
6. Open communication and sharing
7. Flexible leadership and decision making; shared power

8. Flexible membership composition, based on case needs
9. A core of stable membership composition
10. A sense of both group identity and professional identity
11. Ability to negotiate and reach consensus
12. Goal focus and goal clarity
13. Record keeping of meetings: dates, members present, issues discussed, decisions made
14. Attention to both the task and maintenance functions of the team
15. A systems perspective

Group Decision-Making Styles

There are at least four decision-making styles in a group: (1) *default* (no decision), (2) *unilateral* (imposed from above), (3) *majority vote* (most agree), and (4) *consensus* (all agree) (Rubin and Beckhard, 1972).

Although consensus is the ideal outcome, it is important to achieve it fairly. Unfortunately, team decision making in health care settings and elsewhere is often undemocratically influenced by those with more prestige or power. In reality, we live in a society in which the medical professional is accorded a level of prestige and power far exceeding that of any other health care profession (Caputi, 1978). In addition, professional education in all fields is primarily university based, with a reward system that reinforces autonomy and competition rather than cooperation and interdisciplinary education and experience (Lodge, 1974). As a result, members of various health professions enter health care settings with little orientation to or experience with one another (Kane, 1976-1977). Furthermore, in most health care settings, it is the physician who is ultimately responsible for patient outcomes and timely discharge. Thus, in a real sense, the call to interdisciplinary teamwork may be experienced as disorienting (Lonsdale, Webb, and Briggs, 1980:106), and those involved may encounter difficulty in achieving its theoretically ideal process and benefits.

Still, we must persist in efforts to develop professional educational preparation for interdisciplinary teamwork, both in the classroom and in practicum, if we expect to make collaborative practice work (Waugaman, 1994; Casto, 1994).

While health service settings are usually multidisciplinary and sometimes interdisciplinary, there are additional features of health service organizations that can influence social work practice in them. These are explored next.

OTHER ORGANIZATIONAL CONSIDERATIONS

Health service settings are secondary settings of social work practice and professional organizations that sometimes have a dual-authority system. They may be complex organizations that also vary by whether they are public, voluntary, or proprietary and by whether they are sectarian or secular. Government efforts to control the rising cost of health services have brought major changes in professional autonomy, paperwork, and intervention criteria, time frame, and prioritization.

Secondary Settings

Health service settings are examples of *secondary settings* of social work practice because their main function is something other than social work. In this case, the primary function is health service. Thus, social work services in health settings are *auxiliary* (supplementary or supportive) and *ancillary* (subordinate) to the services of the medical and nursing care staff. The obvious exception to this is the community mental health agency, where social workers are among the primary, rather than secondary, service providers.

This does not necessarily mean that social work services are not highly valued by the medical and nursing staff, or that social workers are expected to behave subserviently to them. It simply means that the medical and nursing functions are more central than the social work functions to the operation of the organizational system. The situation would be reversed if, for example, a social work organization, such as a child welfare agency, employed one or more physicians or nurses as consultants to the social work staff or to assess and treat children with physical signs and symptoms of abuse or neglect.

What the secondary-setting nature of health service organizations does imply for social workers who practice in them is that to be accepted by the primary service providers and to be utilized fully and appropriately, social workers must (1) be considerate and respectful of the primary service providers and their work and responsibilities; (2) be mindful of the fact that medical and nursing staff view the patient as "their patient" and will appreciate the social worker keeping them informed of any developments concerning the patient or family; and (3) keep in mind the primary and priority functions of the organization, as well as the associated perspectives and concerns of the primary service providers.

Problems in cooperating with these primary providers usually arise when social workers become too preoccupied with their own work and neglect this *caveat* (warning).

Professional Organizations

Another feature of health service settings is that they are professional organizations, since members of professions are the primary staff. In professional organizations, roles are not firmly defined nor established by the personnel office or the professional group itself, but must be "won" through a kind of political process in which *turf* (domain) is negotiated with other professionals in an ongoing fashion (Bucher and Stelling, 1978).

This means that social workers cannot expect to enter the organization and simply do their job as they envision it from their professional education. Instead, they must be aware that their role definition is dependent on the cooperation and *tacit* (implied) consent of other professionals in the organization, who may or may not perceive their own roles as including some of what social workers think is theirs.

For example, in most hospitals, a main function of social work is *discharge planning*. However, physicians and nurses may see some aspects of discharge planning as part of their own functions. Another example is that social workers tend to think of *psychosocial* problems as a social work arena. Yet, physicians and nurses increasingly perceive psychosocial problems as appropriate to their domain (Cowles and Lefcowitz, 1995).

On the other hand, social workers may obtain information from patients or families that suggests a different diagnosis of the patient's health problem than the physician has assigned. If the social worker shares this information with the attending physician, the physician may be less than enthusiastic and view it as a *turf viola-tion.*

The point is that in professional organizations, each professional is not as *autonomous* (independent) as he or she might be in private practice or in a predominately bureaucratic organization.

Dual-Authority System

An unusual organizational characteristic in hospitals is that two lines of authority often exist: the bureaucratic chain of command and the medical staff chain of command (Coe, 1978; Smith, 1978). Because of the unique authority, autonomy, and responsibility granted to the medical profession, its members do not always con-cur with, or concede to, the rules, regulations, and policies estab-lished by the board of directors or administrators. This means that social workers and other personnel who practice in such settings cannot assume that simply because they are acting in compliance with the official policy of the organization that the medical staff will not sometimes take exception to their actions and demand another course. There is no easy solution to this potential problem. It is simply important to be aware that it exists and to develop sensitivity to the types of situations that might provoke its appearance.

Complex Organizations

Complex organizations are those which provide multiple services or functions and/or have multiple staff positions and roles.

Health service organizations, especially hospitals, are referred to as "complex organizations" because they have a complex division of labor and because they have several functions, which sometimes are subdivided into multiple-service units.

A *complex division of labor* means that the assignment of "who does and is responsible for what" is delegated among multiple personnel. This is not always easy to sort out. There are various positions among medical and nursing staff, and sometimes several layers of personnel in other departments, such as dietary, pharmacy, and physical therapy.

Social workers need to be familiar with this division of labor among the personnel in the organization in which they practice. If they are not clear about it, they are likely to seek information from, or report information to, inappropriate persons.

In addition, especially in hospitals, the organization often has more than one function (i.e., complex functions). Although the primary function is health care service, hospitals have multiple *units of health service,* such as the emergency room, outpatient clinics, and a variety of inpatient service units. The organization may also provide *education* or training for various types of health service professionals and other personnel. *Research* is another common function, especially of large teaching hospitals.

It is important for social workers to be familiar with the functions of the organization itself. First, to develop their own roles in an organization, social workers must know what the organization does. A setting with a professional education function may afford opportunities for social workers to teach students in the program about the social worker perspective of their role in the setting or about the biopsychosocial perspective as it relates to specific types of health problems. Similarly, settings whose functions include research may provide opportunities for social workers to collaborate on research projects. Second, a social worker employed in an organization is a representative of the organization and ought to be able to accurately describe its functions to others. Finally, organizational function is a major determinant of the social worker role in the organization. Although all health service organizations share the common and primary function of providing "health service," the form this function takes, and the function of the social worker, varies with whether the level of intervention is primary, secondary, or tertiary care.

For example, hospitals provide short-term intervention at the secondary level, which limits the length of time the social worker has to work with the patient or family. It also means that much of the time the patient is there, he or she often will be quite ill, which also limits social work intervention with the patient. Thus, for the most part, social and/or emotional problems that the social worker identifies will be referred to outside agencies for service, and the social worker will need to focus on services that support and complement the short-term care objectives of the hospital setting. On the other hand, in a hospice program, the health care service is often of longer duration and focused on supporting the function and comfort of the patient rather than on repairing the health problem. The social worker function is accordingly adapted to enhance this particular organizational function.

Similar differences in the health care functions of rehabilitation centers, nursing homes, and primary care settings exist, which will be discussed further in later chapters.

Funding Sources and the Profit Motive

A variable of health service organizations is the source of their funds and the extent to which they operate for financial profit. There are three main types of organizations with regard to funding source and profit: (1) public, (2) voluntary, and (3) proprietary.

Public organizations are owned and operated by federal, state, or local government, receive the largest share of their funds from public tax support, and are nonprofit. There are many examples of such publicly funded health service organizations, such as VA hospitals, county tax-supported hospitals, state tax-supported general medical and surgical-type hospitals, as well as specialty hospitals such as for the chronically mentally ill or developmentally disabled. The VA also supports some nursing home, home care, and rehabilitation programs. Some counties also support nursing homes, drug and alcohol treatment programs, and day treatment programs for the chronically mentally ill or the impaired elderly, such as patients with Alzheimer's disease. Other examples of public organizations include the federal, state, and county "public health services," which are usually concerned with primary prevention of health problems through controlling communicable diseases, operating prenatal and well-baby clinics, as well as through public education and research.

Voluntary organizations are "private but nonprofit" and often are *sectarian* (affiliated with some religious sect). Examples of such health service organizations include Catholic, Jewish, Lutheran, and Methodist hospitals, nursing homes, and hospice programs. In addition, certain civic organizations, such as the Shriners, Masons, or American Legion, sometimes operate hospitals or nursing home care facilities. Voluntary and other organizations that are not religiously affiliated are called *secular* organizations.

Finally, health service organizations increasingly are *proprietary* ones, which means that they are both privately owned and operated for profit. Of the three types of health service organizations, proprietary organizations are the most rapidly growing type. Examples include the Columbia/HCA (Hospital Corporation of America), the largest nationwide chain of profit-making hospitals; Beverly Enterprises, the largest nationwide nursing home chain; Caremark, the largest chain of home health care agencies; and CIGNA, an insurance company and the largest chain of managed care facilities. In addition, many of the community mental health centers that were originally established as public tax-supported facilities to provide both outpatient and inpatient services for mental health problems, as well as drug and alcohol addiction, have now become private profit-making organizations, such as community psychiatric centers. The number of profit-making home care agencies also has mushroomed in recent years (Karger and Stoesz, 1998:188-191).

The funding source differences among these three types of organizations are growing increasingly difficult to distinguish. The reason is that since the Medicaid and Medicare programs were established in the mid-1960s, an increasing share of funding for all kinds of health services is coming from these tax-supported programs. Whereas Medicare is a federally funded program whose revenue is derived from payroll taxes, Medicaid is both federal and state supported, meaning its funds come from the general revenues of federal and state governments. Today, whether a health service is a public, voluntary, or proprietary facility, a large part of its funds are derived from government-financed programs.

All three types of organizations may obtain a considerable share of their funds from patient *fees for service* (charges that are based on the kind and number of provided services, in contrast to a *prepaid fee system*, whereby a set amount is paid before service, which covers whatever services are later determined to be needed). However, patient fees may be obtained *out of pocket* (fees that the individual pays because he or she lacks insurance coverage for all or part of the service), through private or public insurance programs, or from other tax-supported programs, such as Title XX, an amendment to the Social Security Act.

The issue, then, is whether any significant differences exist among the three types of organizations that are relevant to social work practice in such settings? Little is known from research to answer this question. However, there are many questions, largely about the quality of patient care in for-profit organizations, especially nursing homes and mental health programs.

The following list presents some of those questions. Is there a tendency for proprietary health service organizations to

1. keep direct service staff-to-patient ratio as low as possible?
2. exclude patients needing service but who lack the ability to pay the established rates?
3. adapt length of service to patient ability to continue to pay?
4. rely too heavily on *psychotropic medications* in place of more time-consuming and costly interventions?
5. neglect the needs of those who are less able to advocate for themselves, such as the elderly and chronically impaired, in favor of those who are more demanding?
6. place too much emphasis on "public appearance," in terms of exterior and front entrance decor, relative to the less visible facilities, equipment, and staff needed to rehabilitate patients and support their comfort and function?
7. keep regular full-time staff to a minimum and to rely on part-time or temporary staff from health personnel employment agencies?
8. generously pay certain key administrative and professional staff, but require them to fulfill role expectations that serve the profit objective more than the patient care objective?
9. employ online staff who meet the minimum standards rather than optimal standards and provide compensation and benefits that are minimal?

The theme of these alleged tendencies of proprietary organizations is that they place more importance on *the bottom line* (profit) than on high quality of patient care. If these allegations are true, social workers who practice in proprietary settings may experience constraints on their ability to practice in accordance with the standards, values, and ethics of their profession, in spite of the appeal of some of the "perks" that can accompany positions in these organizations.

The Impact of Medicaid and Medicare

We have already alluded to the rapid growth in the Medicaid and Medicare programs in recent years and the increasing share of health care costs that these programs finance. This development has affected social work practice in health service settings, largely as a result of government efforts to control the cost of health care.

One effect of these cost-control efforts has been a general trend toward limiting social work services reimbursable by the two main government health insurance programs to those which are clearly related to the patient's current health condition and to the health care services being provided for that condition. Another effect has been an increase in organizational paperwork required to document claims for reimbursement. This has led to a corresponding increased rate of error and loss of reimbursement. This fear of not being reimbursed has led to a general tendency to limit services to those which are essential. Since the two government financing programs only reimburse services that are ordered or approved by the physician, this too has acted as a constraint on the provision of social work services.

Finally, federal government efforts to contain the rapid increase in health care costs led to passage of the Tax Equity and Fiscal Responsibility Act in 1983, which established the now familiar DRG (diagnosis-related group) system. This system limits the length of stay of hospitalized patients to a prescribed period of time, depending on the diagnosis. Overstays must be paid by the hospital itself, not the patient. Thus, the overall effect of the DRG system has been earlier release of most patients. This reduction in length of stay has further constrained what the social worker can attempt to do with inpatients and places even greater priority on the social worker function of assisting with arrangements for posthospital continuity of care in a nursing home, home care, or other plan.

Similarly, an increasing percentage of nursing home care is being reimbursed by the government-funded programs, especially for Medicare-eligible persons who need such a setting as an extended care facility following a hospitalization. Often, however, the brief Medicare reimbursable period expires before the patient is ready to be released from the nursing home. This frequently requires the social worker serving the nursing home to assist in finding other sources of reimbursement or to arrange for home care.

SOCIAL WORKER FUNCTIONS AND CLIENT PROBLEMS

Professional Standards for Social Worker Functions

The following is part of a standard set by the National Association of Social Workers regarding social work in health care settings (Standard 4):

> The functions of the social work program shall include specific services to the client population and the community in keeping with the overall mission of the organization. These shall include direct services, consultation, education, policy and program planning, quality assurance, advocacy, and liaison with the community. When the organization assumes teaching and research functions, the social work program should participate in them. Research, social work field instruction, and other teaching responsibilities are appropriate and recommended functions of all social work programs. (NASW, 1987:6)

This standard (NASW, 1987:6-7) interprets the previous statement as follows:

> Specific services to the client population shall include but not be limited to these:
>
> • Assessment of the need for social work services.
> • Preadmission planning and discharge planning.
> • Direct services and treatment to individuals, families, and groups.
> • Case-finding and outreach.
> • Information and referral.

- Client advocacy within and outside the organization, including attention to fiscal constraints.
- Protection of clients' rights and entitlement, including the right to redress.
- Short and long term planning.
- Promotion and maintenance of health and mental health.
- Preventive, remedial, and rehabilitative measures.
- Provision for continuity of care, including guarantee of access and effective utilization.

Services to the community shall include but not be limited to the following:

- Identification of unmet needs and unserved groups.
- Identification of and service to at-risk populations.
- Consultation and collaboration with outside organizations and professionals concerning the care of populations and the promotion of health.
- Community liaison services.
- Community planning and coordination activities.
- Psychosocial health education and promotion.

Since the services to the client population and the community are interrelated and may overlap, the foregoing classifications of functions are not restricted to the particular areas mentioned.

Consultation regarding the social, environmental, psychological, and cultural factors that affect health maintenance should be provided to those involved in the client's care. They may include the agency and its staff, the community, outside agencies and professionals, and significant others.

There are four NASW expectations concerning functions of social workers in health care settings that are particularly important to note: (1) both direct and indirect services should be provided; (2) social workers should reach out to clients who need their services; (3) the primary obligation of social workers is to their clients' rights and needs; and (4) services should be provided, not only to individual clients, but also to families, groups, and the community.

Both Direct and Indirect Services

The first paragraph in the fourth NASW standard clarifies that the core social worker functions in health care settings should include both *direct services* to clients and *indirect services* such as consultation, teaching, research, and program development.

This is important to heed because social workers in health care settings, especially in hospitals, have tended to focus too heavily on direct services and too little on indirect services. Yet, it is research that serves to develop the body of practice knowledge on which the claim to "professionalism" is primarily based, while program development is the mechanism for improving services and other resources for clients, and consultation and teaching are major instruments for promoting social work knowledge, skills, values, and influence.

A major direct-service function of social workers in health care settings is "treatment" of patient problems. It should be noted that social workers do not "treat" physical health problems, except insofar as modification of client attitudes, feelings, behaviors, and so forth, or modification of the environmental situation may serve to improve the client's health. However, in mental health settings, social workers with a master's degree or doctoral degree are often among the major providers of treatment for mental health problems.

Case Finding

The second paragraph in the NASW statement elaborates on the kinds of social work services that should be available to clients in health care settings and includes reference to "assessment of the need for social work services" and "case-finding and outreach."

This is important because it underscores the need for social workers in health care settings to avoid their traditional tendency to rely heavily on referrals from physicians and nurses, which allowed these other groups to select the kinds of client problems the social workers would address.

Primacy of the Clients' Rights and Needs

The references to "client advocacy . . . ," "protection of clients' rights . . . ," and "provision of continuity of care, including provision of access and effective utilization" highlight the need for social workers to remember their primary obligation to the clients' rights and needs and to actively avoid becoming a party either to organizational or other constraints on meeting client needs or to violations of client rights.

Services to All Client Levels

Finally, the reference to "direct services and treatment to individuals, families, and groups," and to specification of "services to the community," implies that the NASW expects social workers in health care settings to work with all "client levels" and, in this sense, to function as generalists rather than specialists.

Health-Related Psychosocial Problems of Clients

The NASW standard for social worker functions in health care settings reflects the kinds of problems often addressed by social workers when working with patients and their families, including (1) barriers to admission to the service or facility; (2) problems of adjustment to the service or facility; (3) problems of adjustment to the diagnosis, prognosis, or health care plan; (4) lack of information to make informed decisions and to feel in control; (5) lack of resources to meet needs; and (6) barriers to discharge from the service or facility.

Barriers to Admission

First, patients sometimes experience *barriers to admission,* that is, conditions that prevent the person from receiving a needed health service. Such barriers may be psychological, financial, informational, or related to family care, transportation, or other concerns or resource needs.

Examples of *psychological barriers* include fear of being admitted to a hospital, nursing home, or other residential care facility, feeling embarrassed to seek help for mental or certain physical health problems, and avoiding having diagnostic tests done for fear of pain, side effects, or the findings.

Financial barriers can include lacking adequate health insurance to cover the anticipated costs of the services, fearing the loss of a job due to time off from work, and worrying about accumulating debt due to a temporary loss of income.

Informational barriers to admission tend to include both lack of enough information and misinformation, for example, uncertainty about what the service experience will be like or having heard rumors or read stories about "terrible things that could happen."

In addition, patients sometimes have other practical concerns such as who will take care of their family, pets, or house while they are an inpatient, not having any transportation to an outpatient service, or having their work accumulate because of missed time.

Most such barriers revolve around social environmental and/or emotional situations or concerns, so assistance with preadmission planning is an appropriate function of social workers.

Adjusting to the Setting or Service

Problems of adjustment to the service or setting are difficulties experienced by the patient or family in feeling comfortable and satisfied with the inpatient or outpatient health service or setting.

Institutional settings, such as hospitals, residential treatment centers, and nursing homes, tend to strip a person of their usual supports (Goffman, 1961), that is, things on which people have come to depend. Such customary supports may include family, friends, familiar places and furnishings, familiar location of things one relies on, freedom to make personal decisions, familiar daily routines, activities, and favorite foods. Most of us are not aware of how dependent we are on these things until we are required to be separated from them.

As a result of these and other situational changes, inpatients can experience an uncomfortable sense of loss of control over their own lives. Residents of such facilities react in various ways to such changes; some adapt with little apparent difficulty, while others withdraw (sometimes to the point of losing touch with reality) or become hostile and defiant, and some even try to leave, and sometimes succeed.

If not resolved through preadmission planning, inpatients of hospitals or nursing homes can also have realistic concerns about what may be happening to their family members, pets, homes, work situations, or unpaid bills in their absence. In addition, both in-patients and outpatients are sometimes concerned, justifiably or not, about the quality of care they receive through the health service. These and similar problems of adaption to the health service or setting are often well understood and dealt with by social workers.

Adjusting to the Diagnosis, Prognosis, or Treatment Plan

Another common problem of patients and/or their family members concerns their coping with the diagnosis, prognosis, or treatment plan. Probably the most difficult adjustment is presented when the diagnosis, prognosis, or treatment plan indicates a likelihood or possibility of impending death.

However, more often the diagnosis, prognosis, or treatment plan has implications for "living with" temporary losses of comfort and function or with *chronic* (ongoing) disabilities that may involve discomfort; functional incapacities; changes in role responsibilities and relationships; disfigurement; dependency on medications, pros-theses, or machines; dietary restrictions; altering lifestyle habits such as drinking, smoking, exercise, and hobbies; or the need for significant changes in the home environment, such as ramps, grab bars, changes in floor coverings, width of doorways, or height of cabinets and light fixtures.

In short, oftentimes, the diagnosis, prognosis, or treatment plan requires major changes in the lives of patients and their family members. The effects usually are both emotional and social envi-ronmental. For example, patients who learn they have a health problem that will require them to quit working or change the nature of their work may face both economic problems and emotional reactions. Patients who learn they will require nursing home care may need to make practical decisions about their homes and fami-lies, but also usually experience feelings of distress about such life changes. Patients who are permanently paralyzed from the waist down face not only a multitude of practical problems concerning how they will function, but also must deal with emotional issues concerning, for example, self-image, sexual relationships, and fears of dependency. Patients who have permanent and severe kidney damage that will require dialysis several hours a week on different days encounter practical problems and often experience accompanying emotional responses to dependency on machinery for survival. These are examples of what are termed "psychosocial" problems because they have both emotional and social environmental components. Such problems are well-suited to the competency preparation of professional social workers.

Need for Information to Make Informed Decisions and Take Control

Another common problem of patients and their family members in health care settings is a sense of diminished control. Actions are planned and sometimes carried out without adequate patient forewarning, explanation, or consent, whether by physicians, nurses, nurse aides, or other staff. The effect can be to provoke a sense of helplessness that compounds problems they may already have in adjusting to the setting or service.

This sense of loss of control is of particular significance in health care settings because, as considerable research evidence suggests, it can lead to depression and "giving up," which in turn tend to negatively impact on optimal comfort, function, and even recovery (Schmale, 1972; Levy, 1974). In short, when people feel a loss of control over their life situations, they may "quit trying." Although the biochemical process is not clearly understood, there is indication that such an emotional response may affect the immune system and other physiological systems that play a role in health status and life expectancy.

The social worker can play an important role by providing appropriate information to patients and their families to assist them in making informed decisions about matters that concern them. When the information they require is clearly the responsibility of the physician or nurse to provide, the social worker can act in the role of a mediator or liaison to bridge the gap between them.

Social workers also assist patients and family members in thinking through their options—whether it involves a proposed medical procedure, the location and type of their posthospital care, or choice of resources to assist them in dealing with the patients' health problem.

Finally, social workers need to advocate for the patients' right to know the facts about their options, to assure their clients that they have this right, and to support clients in claiming it.

Lack of Resources to Meet Needs

Probably no function in health care settings is more appreciated by patients and families, as well as by physicians and nurses, than for social workers to assist patients and their families in obtaining resources to help meet patients' health care needs. Such resources usually fall into five categories: (1) medical aids and appliances, (2) income supports, (3) services, (4) environmental adaptations, and (5) interpersonal supports.

Medical aids and appliances, or tools and equipment, can encompass a range of items such as wheelchairs, walkers, canes, grab bars, raised toilet seats, portable commodes, long-handled prongs for reaching, eyeglasses, hearing aids, hospital beds, geri-chairs, cardiac chairs, alternating air pressure mattresses, suction machines, blood sugar testing kits, blood pressure cuffs, incontinence pads, Hoya-lifts, gel-filled chair pads, corrective shoes, or braces. The need for such equipment is usually associated with home care situations, although there are occasions when patients in hospitals or nursing care facilities need special equipment that is not furnished by the facility.

Support services are also widely varied. Those most often required in the field of health care include the following: (1) personal care services (assistance with activities of daily living, such as bathing, feeding, dressing, grooming, excretion), which may be provided by family members, home care agencies, or independent nursing assistants; (2) professional nursing services (for example, wound care, monitoring vital signs, catheter changes, and i.v. regulation, often provided by visiting nurse services associated with or independent of a home care agency; (3) physical therapy; (4) housekeeping services; (5) transportation services for the elderly and handicapped; (6) home-delivered meal services; (7) family counseling services; (8) drug and alcohol treatment services; (9) hospice care programs; (10) telephone reassurance services; (11) lifeline services; (12) adult or child protection services; (13) respite-care services; (14) day care; (15) foreign language interpreter services; and (16) vocational retraining.

Income support is a major area of resources often needed by patients and their families. Frequently, the need for income assistance is associated with paying for the health care service agency itself, whether outpatient care, hospitalization, nursing home care, home care, day care agency services, or hospice program services. In addition, income assistance is often needed to pay for medical aids and appliances and many of the various services previously listed. Furthermore, patients in health care settings are sometimes found to lack resources to support basic living needs, such as adequate housing and food, without which their health is further threatened.

Income supports generally come in two main forms: cash or in-kind. *Cash income supports are economic assistance received in cash/checks to be used as needed.* Examples of cash income assistance include Social Security, Supplemental Security Income, Temporary Aid to Families with Children, Veteran's Pensions, Unemployment Compensation, Workmen's Compensation, and General Assistance (which in some states is provided through the township trustees). On the other hand, *in-kind income supports are economic assistance that is received, not in cash, but in the form of the service or resource needed* (e.g., food, clothing, housing, medical care). Examples of in-kind income support programs include Medicare, Medicaid, public housing, subsidized private housing, food stamps, food and clothing bank programs, and shelters for the homeless. Whereas cash income support programs provide benefits in the form of checks for clients to cash and use to purchase what they need, in-kind income support programs pay the service provider directly or provide clients with the material object itself, instead of cash to purchase it, or with a voucher that can be traded only for the specified commodity.

Environmental adaptations are important resources for persons who have mental or physical disabilities that require certain changes in the setting around them in order to be able to function as well as possible. For the physically impaired, these may include ramps, wide doorways to accommodate wheelchairs, rearrangement of furnishings to make them reachable, nonskid floors, or low-pile carpets. Depending on the type of mental impairment, helpful environmental adaptations could include a fenced-in yard (to prevent wandering), low-level sounds, avoidance of interpersonal conflicts, simplicity and sameness of furnishings, or strategically placed labels to help locate vital areas.

Interpersonal supports are needed by most people. These involve having ready access to other people who provide human relationships and social interactions that are experienced as emotionally supportive (feeling held up), including feeling cared about and valued. Having such interpersonal support is a fundamental human need and plays a vital role at all levels of health care service.

Barriers to Discharge

Patient and family *barriers to discharge* are things that prevent patients from terminating their inpatient or outpatient services once they are ready for release. Such barriers are similar to barriers to admission to health care services; that is, they may be psychological, financial, informational, or related to family care, transportation, or other concerns or resource needs.

A psychological barrier to discharge could be that the patient has grown emotionally dependent on the service and fears being separated from it. A financial barrier to discharge could be that the patient has no income and no place to go after discharge. An informational barrier to discharge could be that the patient does not know enough about nursing homes or home care agencies to make arrangements for such services. An example of a family care barrier to discharge is that a patient may need extended care in another facility but does not know how his or her family would manage for such a prolonged absence. Finally, the patient may simply have no way to travel from the inpatient location to the next service location and may require assistance in arranging for transportation and/or paying for it.

In many instances, hospitalized patients and/or their family members are fully able to handle the release and aftercare without professional assistance. However, this is not always the case.

Patients usually need assistance with discharge planning when (1) their health condition at the expected time of release is such that they will require some kind of assistance afterward; (2) it is not clear to the medical or nursing staff what resources patients have at home to manage their aftercare; (3) the patients or families need information about, and assistance in, making arrangements for nursing homes, home care, or hospice care programs; and (4) the patients or families need assistance in identifying their options and making decisions concerning their choice of aftercare.

It is important to understand that when social workers help with these various types of problems, services are, oftentimes, but not always, directed to individual patients and individual family members. Social workers also sometimes relate to all or several members of a family together, or to a group of patients or families with similar problems or needs—whether to provide information, orientation, instruction, or some sort of counseling or problem solving.

In addition, in the course of serving clients in these direct ways, social workers sometimes identify gaps in community resources for certain types of client needs, or they may identify some unhealthy condition in a community that needs to be corrected to reduce the future incidence of problems such as those faced by their clients. Thus, social workers may need to become involved in what is variously called community organization, social action, and policy/program planning and development. Such community-directed services, along with teaching, research, and consultation, are termed "indirect services" because they are not provided to clients, but on behalf of clients.

It should also be remembered that the need for improved resources or environmental changes, calling for policy/program planning and development, may be within the health service itself. Social workers are often in a unique position to learn from clients what is problematic about the service or facility itself, as clients often more readily share such information with social workers than with physicians or nurses. Social workers have a responsibility to try to help improve the quality and delivery of services in the setting where they practice.

The next chapter discusses the knowledge, values and ethics, skills and interventions of social workers in health service settings.

SUMMARY

Since the beginning of social work in health care in the general hospital setting in 1905, its practitioners have seen their role as complementing the functions of the medical and nursing staff by addressing the problematic social, environmental, and psychological experiences of the patient and family that accompany the patient's health condition and its treatment. Currently, about 52 percent of NASW members primarily practice in the health field, in mental and physical health programs combined, while about 38 percent of NASW members are located primarily in mental or physical health organizational settings.

The underlying theoretical perspective of social work in the health field is that biological, psychological, and social systems reciprocally influence one another as causes and effects of health problems. While "medical care" is what physicians provide in their efforts to monitor patient health and to treat health problems, social work practice in the health field is addressed to the individual attitudes, behaviors, and social environmental resources of people that are vital to "health care" at the three levels of prevention, remediation, and compensation.

What people do, or do not do, to take care of their own health, how people interpret and respond to what could be symptoms of health problems, and how people behave after they are determined to be ill or injured are complex phenomena that reflect multiple human diversity variables. There is a body of knowledge about broad differences in human behavior associated with, for example, gender, ethnicity, socioeconomic class, and age. However, such knowledge cannot predict how particular individuals will behave given their combined characteristics.

Most health service settings employ a multidisciplinary staff. Sometimes, such settings utilize "interdisciplinary" teams to assess and intervene in health care. The mission of such teams is to coordinate comprehensive services addressed to the often multiple and interdependent problems of the "whole patient" in an effort to enhance the success of services and to reduce gaps and overlap in services. Although information is available regarding the functions, requirements, and problems of interdisciplinary teams, unfortunately, most professional education does not adequately prepare workers for this type of group practice.

Health service organizations are secondary settings of social work, and they are professional rather than typical bureaucratic organizations. In those settings with physician-dominated health services, such as hospitals, there may be a dual-authority system, that is, both a bureaucratic and a physician chain of command that run parallel to each other. In addition, health service organizations such as hospitals, community mental health centers, and public health agencies often have a complex division of labor and/or complex functions, and thus are called complex organizations.

Health service organizations also vary by whether they are public, voluntary, or proprietary ones and by whether they are sectarian or secular. Proprietary health service organizations are the most rapidly growing type, and considerable concern has been expressed about the alleged impact of a financial profit incentive on the quality of health services.

Finally, as the increased cost of health services has become recognized as one of our nation's most serious social problems, cost-containment efforts of government health care financing programs have intensified in ways that include effects on social work in health services.

Thus, a variety of characteristics of health service organizations tends to constrain the role and function of the social workers who practice in them. The challenge for social workers is to find ways to adapt that will maximize their efficiency and effectiveness for the sake of all concerned—patient and family, organization, and funding source.

The basic and essential functions of social workers in health service settings include direct services *to patients and families*, individually or in small groups, as well as the functions of consultation, education, policy and program planning, quality assurance, advocacy, *and* liaison with the *community*. Recommended functions of social workers in the health field include research, social work field instruction, and other teaching.

Chapter 2

Fundamentals of Health Care Social Work Practice

KNOWLEDGE REQUIREMENTS

The Knowledge Base of Professionalism

The basic characteristic that distinguishes a profession from simply an occupation is that a profession lays claim to, "professes" to have, a body of knowledge on which its members base their practice of service to others. The specialized nature of this knowledge leads people outside the profession to view a member of the profession as "an authority" in the knowledge area and to grant the profession "the authority" to practice with little interference from outsiders, that is, autonomy of practice (Greenwood, 1957). This body of professional knowledge is expected to be sufficiently extensive and complex that preparation for entrance to the profession requires a lengthy educational process, which is usually university based.

Definition of the Social Work Profession

Social work has been defined as the *professional* activity of helping individuals, families, groups, or communities to enhance or restore their capacity for social functioning and of creating societal conditions favorable to this goal (NASW, 1991). Thus, as a profession, social work claims to have special knowledge and skills that better qualify its members, as opposed to nonmembers, to provide such helping services.

The Meaning of Knowledge

For centuries, philosophers, theologians, scientists, and members of other disciplines have debated about what constitutes "knowledge." Much of their debate revolves around the issue of the *process* through which knowledge is obtained. Philosophy and theology are prescientific or extrascientific fields because they predate science and adhere to processes of "knowing," such as logical deduction and religious experience, which are outside the process of modern science. For the most part, professions, including social work, uphold the *scientific* process of developing knowledge, which emphasizes the importance of *unbiased observation* (objectivity) and theory building.

Knowledge As Theory

In the realm of science, knowledge is not mere fact finding, such as might be performed through a population census, an opinion poll, or other modes of observing phenomena. Instead, such gathered facts or pieces of information need to be related to explanations of what the facts mean, of how they are related to each other or to other facts (Wing, 1978). Preliminary or tentative explanations are called *hypotheses*. As hypotheses are tested and found to be supported or not, a body of *theory* (explanation) is developed; this is called knowledge. Such knowledge or theory is never final or complete, but is always open to modification as additional research gathers new evidence.

One concession that science perhaps owes to other more intuitive approaches to knowledge is that much of scientific development begins with *casual observations*, or "hunches," about some aspect of reality. That is, before people formulate a hypothesis about something, they usually "happened to notice something," or "got an idea that . . ." Often this occurs in the course of everyday experience, or, in professions, in the course of practice experience. In the latter case, we call these *practice hunches*, or pieces of practice wisdom. Often, such hunches are the "seeds" of knowledge development, in that they may be used to formulate a research question, which is the first step in the scientific process.

The Scientific Process

In all science, a particular process is required. Although the initial stimulus may be only a "hunch" about some aspect of reality, the scientific process involves a series of particular steps (Neuman, 1994:11):

1. Formulate a research question.
2. Review the literature.
3. Refine the research question.
4. Design a plan for researching that question, including
   a. sampling,
   b. data collection, and
   c. data analysis.
5. Conduct the study.
6. Analyze the data to draw conclusions regarding the research question.
7. Disseminate the findings to others.

As noted earlier, a "hunch," or *piece of practice wisdom*, is often the basis for formulating a research question, such as "Is the poverty rate correlated with the reported child abuse rate?" or "Does the level of patient participation in discharge planning affect patients' likelihood of relapse?" Such research questions are then explored through reading about previous studies of the issue to determine what their findings and conclusions have been. Based on these, the research question is refined and/or simply translated into a hypothesis, such as "As the poverty rate increases in a population, the reported child abuse rate increases," or "The less patient involvement in discharge planning, the earlier patients relapse." The hypothesis is then tested through the research process, and the findings are disseminated through professional journals, adding to the cumulative *body of knowledge* (theory) on the subject.

In summary, a profession must have a body of knowledge that justifies its authority to practice. Scientific knowledge is theory building through a specific process that helps to (1) ensure that each new study builds on previous ones and (2) forces researchers to think through how they will address the particular research question beforehand to determine whether or not the issue can be researched.

Generic Social Work Knowledge Areas

Social work education programs revolve around four core knowledge areas that are considered essential for all social work, regardless of client population, field of practice, or setting. These generic areas of social work knowledge are as follows:

1. *Human behavior and the social environment:* an integration of scientific theory about the role of biological, psychological, and sociocultural factors in human behavior and development.
2. *Social welfare policy and programs:* knowledge of the historical development and current features of social welfare programs and policies in society to address social problems—including community resources available to help people, gaps in resources, the process of policy/program development in society, and how social workers can influence such development.
3. *Social work practice:* theory concerning the social work helping process, methods of social work practice, skills, techniques, and intervention modalities, as well as the values and ethics of professional social work practice.
4. *Research Methods:* knowledge of the scientific research process, both quantitative and qualitative, principles and methods of sampling, data collection, and data analysis that are suited to social work practice.

Of these four knowledge areas, number 3 is uniquely social work knowledge—social work practice knowledge. It is this knowledge that needs ongoing development so that social work can maintain its status as a profession.

Because social workers address such a broad range of human problems and often practice in a variety of fields and practice settings in the course of their careers, the additional knowledge needed for effective practice with particular client populations, fields, and settings is acquired largely through continuing education, both formal and informal, often while working in the setting.

Health Field-Specific Knowledge Areas

Similarly, social work practice within the health field varies somewhat with the particular client population, problem area, organizational setting, and community context of practice; it will therefore be helpful if the social worker has additional knowledge of the following:

1. *Client population and problem area:* the characteristics of the client population, the nature of the health problem(s) dealt with in the setting, and the common path, treatment, or management of the disorder(s); the biopsychosocial perspective of these disorders; the role of human diversity in the onset and course of the disorders and influence on (a) health behavior, (b) illness behavior, and (c) sick-role behavior. Inevitably, this type of knowledge involves acquiring some additional vocabulary, often medical and psychiatric terms.

2. *Organizational setting:* the characteristics of the organizational setting and their implications for social work, such as whether it is for-profit or nonprofit; secular or sectarian; its mission and function(s); level of health service intervention; authority structure; the types of health professions and occupations in the setting and their roles and role expectations of social work; organizational policy, rules and regulations; and interdisciplinary teamwork principles and practice problems.

3. *Community and its resources:* the characteristics of the surrounding community, such as rural/urban/suburban, population demographics, political attitudes, major business and industry, as well as the resources of that community, including general resources and those of special relevance to the needs of the client population and problem area served by the practice setting.

4. *Specific intervention modalities:* approaches tailored to the needs of the particular client population, problem area, and organizational characteristics, such as crisis intervention, grief counseling, behavioral modification, or case management.

5. *Research, evaluation, and documentation:* the findings and methods of research, evaluation, and documentation that are appropriate to and/or required by the practice setting.

The Relationship Between Generic and Specific Knowledge

The special knowledge required for practice in the health field is not "different" from generic social work knowledge; it is a more in-depth development or specialized understanding of certain aspects of it.

Knowledge of the *particular client population and problem area* in the context of the biopsychosocial model and human diversity and knowledge of community characteristics are in-depth developments of generic knowledge of human behavior and the social environment. Knowledge of the *organizational setting and community resources* is a development of general knowledge of social welfare policy and programs. Although all social workers gain some introduction to and overview of a range of *intervention modalities* in social work practice during their basic professional education, practice in a specific setting usually requires development of knowledge of particular interventions that are most appropriate in that setting. Finally, knowledge of appropriate *research, evaluation, and documentation* useful to and/or required in the setting is a development of basic social work research methods.

In short, generic social work knowledge is the foundation upon which all social work practice is based. Social work practice in the health field, or in any other field, simply requires further development of this basic knowledge in ways that are specific to the clientele, problems, organization, and community of the particular practice setting.

VALUES AND ETHICS CONSIDERATIONS

The Values Base of Professionalism

In addition to a knowledge base, a profession must have a code of ethics that reflects the underlying values of the profession and delineates its standards for the professional behavior of its members. The rationale for this is that since a profession is granted relative autonomy from outside supervision, it must assume responsibility for regulating its own members.

The Meaning of Values and Ethics

Values are what one regards as important or worthwhile. *Ethics* are behavioral norms. A *code of ethics* is a set of behavioral expectations, that is, norms.

The Relationship Between Values and Ethics

Ethics usually reflect our underlying values. What we consider *appropriate behavior* (proper to the situation) tends to reflect what we view to be important or worthwhile.

The Basic Values and Practice Principles of the Social Work Profession

Ethical Principles

The following broad ethical principles are based on social work's core values of service, social justice, dignity and worth of the person, importance of human relationships, integrity, and competence. These principles set forth ideals to which all social workers should aspire.

Value: *Service*

Ethical Principle: *Social workers' primary goal is to help people in need and to address social problems.*

Social workers elevate service to others above self-interest. Social workers draw on their knowledge, values, and skills to help people in need and to address social problems. Social workers are encouraged to volunteer some portion of their professional skills with no expectation of significant financial return (pro bono service).

Value: *Social Justice*

Ethical Principle: *Social workers challenge social injustice.*

Social workers pursue social change, particularly with and on behalf of vulnerable and oppressed individuals and groups of people.

Social workers' social change efforts are focused primarily on issues of poverty, unemployment, discrimination, and other forms of social injustice. These activities seek to promote sensitivity to and knowledge about oppression and cultural and ethnic diversity. Social workers strive to ensure access to needed information, services, and resources; equality of opportunity; and meaningful participation in decision making for all people.

Value: *Dignity and Worth of the Person*

Ethical Principle: *Social workers respect the inherent dignity and worth of the person.*

Social workers treat each person in a caring and respectful fashion, mindful of individual differences and cultural and ethnic diversity. Social workers promote clients' socially responsible self-determination. Social workers seek to enhance clients' capacity and opportunity to change and to address their own needs. Social workers are cognizant of their dual responsibility to clients and to the broader society. They seek to resolve conflicts between clients' interests and the broader society's interests in a socially responsible manner consistent with the values, ethical principles, and ethical standards of the profession.

Value: *Importance of Human Relationships*

Ethical Principle: *Social workers recognize the central importance of human relationships.*

Social workers understand that relationships between and among people are an important vehicle for change. Social workers engage people as partners in the helping process. Social workers seek to strengthen relationships among people in a purposeful effort to promote, restore, maintain, and enhance the well-being of individuals, families, social groups, organizations, and communities.

Value: *Integrity*

Ethical Principle: *Social workers behave in a trustworthy manner.*

Social workers are continually aware of the profession's mission, values, ethical principles, and ethical standards and practice in a manner consistent with them. Social workers act honestly and responsibly and promote ethical practices on the part of the organizations with which they are affiliated.

Value: *Competence*

Ethical Principle: *Social workers practice within their areas of competence and develop and enhance their professional expertise.*

Social workers continually strive to increase their professional knowledge and skills and to apply them in practice. Social workers should aspire to contribute to the knowledge base of the profession. (NASW, 1996:5-6)

Ethical Standards of Professional Social Work Practice

Ethical Standards

1. SOCIAL WORKERS' ETHICAL RESPONSIBILITIES TO CLIENTS

1.01 Commitment to Clients
Social workers' primary responsibility is to promote the well-being of clients. In general, clients' interests are primary. However, social workers' responsibility to the larger society or specific legal obligations may on limited occasions supersede the loyalty owed clients, and clients should be so advised. (Examples include when a social worker is required by law to report that a client has abused a child or has threatened to harm self or others.)

1.02 Self-Determination
Social workers respect and promote the right of clients to self-determination and assist clients in their efforts to identify and clarify their goals. Social workers may limit clients' right to self-determination when, in the social workers' professional judgment, clients' actions or potential actions pose a serious, foreseeable, and imminent risk to themselves or others.

1.03 Informed Consent

(a) Social workers should provide services to clients only in the context of a professional relationship based, when appropriate, on valid informed consent. Social workers should use clear and understandable language to inform clients of the purpose of the services, risks related to the services, limits to services because of the requirements of a third-party payer, relevant costs, reasonable alternatives, clients' right to refuse or withdraw consent, and the time frame covered by the consent. Social workers should provide clients with an opportunity to ask questions.

(b) In instances when clients are not literate or have difficulty understanding the primary language used in the practice setting, social workers should take steps to ensure clients' comprehension. This may include providing clients with a detailed verbal explanation or arranging for a qualified interpreter or translator whenever possible.

(c) In instances when clients lack the capacity to provide informed consent, social workers should protect clients' interests by seeking permission from an appropriate third party, informing clients consistent with the clients' level of understanding. In such instances social workers should seek to ensure that the third party acts in a manner consistent with clients' wishes and interests. Social workers should take reasonable steps to enhance such clients' ability to give informed consent.

(d) In instances when clients are receiving services involuntarily, social workers should provide information about the nature and extent of services and about the extent of clients' right to refuse service.

(e) Social workers who provide services via electronic media (such as computer, telephone, radio, and television) should inform recipients of the limitations and risks associated with such services.

(f) Social workers should obtain clients' informed consent before audiotaping or videotaping clients or permitting observation of services to clients by a third party.

1.04 Competence

(a) Social workers should provide services and represent themselves as competent only within the boundaries of their education, training, license, certification, consultation received, supervised experience, or other relevant professional experience.

(b) Social workers should provide services in substantive areas or use intervention techniques or approaches that are new to them only after engaging in appropriate study, training, consultation, and supervision from people who are competent in those interventions or techniques.

(c) When generally recognized standards do not exist with respect to an emerging area of practice, social workers should exercise careful judgment and take responsible steps (including appropriate education, research, training, consultation, and supervision) to ensure the competence of their work and to protect clients from harm.

1.05 Cultural Competence and Social Diversity

(a) Social workers should understand culture and its function in human behavior and society, recognizing the strengths that exist in all cultures.

(b) Social workers should have a knowledge base of their clients' cultures and be able to demonstrate competence in the provision of services that are sensitive to clients' cultures and to differences among people and cultural groups.

(c) Social workers should obtain education about and seek to understand the nature of social diversity and oppression with respect to race, ethnicity, national origin, color, sex, sexual orientation, age, marital status, political belief, religion, and mental or physical disability.

1.06 Conflicts of Interest

(a) Social workers should be alert to and avoid conflicts of interest that interfere with the exercise of professional discretion and impartial judgment. Social workers should inform clients when a real or potential conflict of interest arises and take reasonable steps to resolve the issue in a manner that makes the clients' interests primary and protects clients' interests to the greatest extent possible. In some cases, protecting clients' interests may require termination of the professional relationship with proper referral of the client.

(b) Social workers should not take unfair advantage of any professional relationship or exploit others to further their personal, religious, political, or business interests.

(c) Social workers should not engage in dual or multiple relationships with clients or former clients in which there is a risk of exploitation or potential harm to the client. In instances when dual or multiple relationships are unavoidable, social workers should take steps to protect clients and are responsible for setting clear, appropriate, and culturally sensitive boundaries. (Dual or multiple relationships occur when social workers relate to clients in more than one relationship, whether professional, social, or business. Dual or multiple relationships can occur simultaneously or consecutively.)

(d) When social workers provide services to two or more people who have a relationship with each other (for example, couples, family members), social workers should clarify with all parties which individuals will be considered clients and the nature of social workers' professional obligations to the various individuals who are receiving services. Social workers who anticipate a conflict of interest among the individuals receiving services or who anticipate having to perform in potentially conflicting roles (for example, when a social worker is asked to testify in a child custody dispute or divorce proceedings involving clients) should clarify their role with the parties involved and take appropriate action to minimize any conflict of interest.

1.07 Privacy and Confidentiality

(a) Social workers should respect clients' right to privacy. Social workers should not solicit private information from clients unless it is essential to providing services or conducting social work evaluation or research. Once private information is shared, standards of confidentiality apply.

(b) Social workers may disclose confidential information when appropriate with valid consent from a client or a person legally authorized to consent on behalf of a client.

(c) Social workers should protect the confidentiality of all information obtained in the course of professional service, except for compelling professional reasons. The general expectation that social workers will keep information confidential does not apply when disclosure is necessary to prevent serious, foreseeable, and imminent harm to a client or other identifiable person or when laws or regulations require disclosure without a client's consent. In all instances, social workers should disclose the least amount of confidential information necessary to achieve the desired purpose; only information that is directly relevant to the purpose for which the disclosure is made should be revealed.

(d) Social workers should inform clients, to the extent possible, about the disclosure of confidential information and the potential consequences, when feasible before the disclosure is made. This applies whether social workers disclose confidential information on the basis of a legal requirement or client consent.

(e) Social workers should discuss with clients and other interested parties the nature of confidentiality and limitations of clients' right to confidentiality. Social workers should review with clients circumstances where confidential information may be requested and where disclosure of confidential information may be legally required. This discussion should occur as soon as possible in the social worker-client relationship and as needed throughout the course of the relationship.

(f) When social workers provide counseling services to families, couples, or groups, social workers should seek agreement among the parties involved concerning each individual's right to confidentiality and obligation to preserve the confidentiality of information shared by others. Social workers should inform participants in family, couples, or group counseling that social workers cannot guarantee that all participants will honor such agreements.

(g) Social workers should inform clients involved in family, couples, marital, or group counseling of the social worker's, employers, and agency's policy concerning the social worker's disclosure of confidential information among the parties involved in the counseling.

(h) Social workers should not disclose confidential information to third-party payers unless clients have authorized such disclosure.

(i) Social workers should not discuss confidential information in any setting unless privacy can be ensured. Social workers should not discuss confidential information in public or semi-public areas such as hallways, waiting rooms, elevators, and restaurants.

(j) Social workers should protect the confidentiality of clients during legal proceedings to the extent permitted by law. When a court of law or other legally authorized body orders social workers to disclose confidential or privileged information without a client's consent and such disclosure could cause harm to the client, social workers should request that the court withdraw the order or limit the order as narrowly as possible or maintain the records under seal, unavailable for public inspection.

(k) Social workers should protect the confidentiality of clients when responding to requests from members of the media.

(l) Social workers should protect the confidentiality of clients' written and electronic records and other sensitive information. Social workers should take reasonable steps to ensure that clients' records are stored in a secure location and that clients' records are not available to others who are not authorized to have access.

(m) Social workers should take precautions to ensure and maintain the confidentiality of information transmitted to other parties through the use of computers, electronic mail, facsimile machines, telephones and telephone answering machines, and other electronic or computer technology. Disclosure of identifying information should be avoided whenever possible.

(n) Social workers should transfer or dispose of clients' records in a manner that protects clients' confidentiality and is consistent with state statutes governing records and social work licensure.

(o) Social workers should take reasonable precautions to protect client confidentiality in the event of the social worker's termination of practice, incapacitation, or death.

(p) Social workers should not disclose identifying information when discussing clients for teaching or training purposes unless the client has consented to disclosure of confidential information.

(q) Social workers should not disclose identifying information when discussing clients with consultants unless the client has consented to disclosure of confidential information or there is a compelling need for such disclosure.

(r) Social workers should protect the confidentiality of deceased clients consistent with the preceding standards.

1.08 Access to Records

(a) Social workers should provide clients with reasonable access to records concerning the clients. Social workers who are concerned that clients' access to their records could cause serious misunderstanding or harm to the client should provide assistance in interpreting the records and consultation with the client regarding the records. Social workers should limit clients' access to their records, or portions of their records, only in exceptional circumstances when there is compelling evidence that such access would cause serious harm to the client. Both clients' requests and the rationale for withholding some or all of the record should be documented in clients' files.

(b) When providing clients with access to their records, social workers should take steps to protect the confidentiality of other individuals identified or discussed in such records.

1.09 Sexual Relationships

(a) Social workers should under no circumstances engage in sexual activities or sexual contact with current clients, whether such contact is consensual or forced.

(b) Social workers should not engage in sexual activities or sexual contact with clients' relatives or other individuals with whom clients maintain a close personal relationship when there is a risk of exploitation or potential harm to the client. Sexual activity or sexual contact with clients' relatives or other individuals with whom clients maintain a personal relationship has the potential to be harmful to the client and may make it difficult for the social worker and client to maintain appropriate professional boundaries. Social workers—not their clients, their clients' relatives, or other individuals with whom the client maintains a personal relationship—assume the full burden for setting clear, appropriate, and culturally sensitive boundaries.

(c) Social workers should not engage in sexual activities or sexual contact with former clients because of the potential for harm to the client. If social workers engage in conduct contrary to this prohibition or claim that an exception to this prohibition is warranted because of extraordinary circumstances, it is social workers—not their clients—who assume the full burden of demonstrating that the former client has not been exploited, coerced, or manipulated, intentionally or unintentionally.

(d) Social workers should not provide clinical services to individuals with whom they have had a prior sexual relationship. Providing clinical services to a former sexual partner has the potential to be harmful to the individual and is likely to make it difficult for the social worker and individual to maintain appropriate professional boundaries.

1.10 Physical Contact

Social workers should not engage in physical contact with clients when there is a possibility of psychological harm to the client as a result of the contact (such as cradling or caressing clients). Social workers who engage in appropriate physical contact with clients are responsible for setting clear, appropriate, and culturally sensitive boundaries that govern such physical contact.

1.11 Sexual Harassment
Social workers should not sexually harass clients. Sexual harassment includes sexual advances, sexual solicitation, requests for sexual favors, and other verbal or physical conduct of a sexual nature.

1.12 Derogatory Language
Social workers should not use derogatory language in their written or verbal communications to or about clients. Social workers should use accurate and respectful language in all communications to and about clients.

1.13 Payment for Services
(a) When setting fees, social workers should ensure that the fees are fair, reasonable, and commensurate with the services performed. Consideration should be given to clients' ability to pay.

(b) Social workers should avoid accepting goods or services from clients as payment for professional services. Bartering arrangements, particularly involving services, create the potential for conflicts of interest, exploitation, and inappropriate boundaries in social workers' relationships with clients. Social workers should explore and may participate in bartering only in very limited circumstances when it can be demonstrated that such arrangements are an accepted practice among professionals in the local community, considered to be essential for the provision of services, negotiated without coercion, and entered into at the client's initiative and with the client's informed consent. Social workers who accept goods or services from clients as payment for professional services assume the full burden of demonstrating that this arrangement will not be detrimental to the client or the professional relationship.

(c) Social workers should not solicit a private fee or other remuneration for providing services to clients who are entitled to such available services through the social workers' employer or agency.

1.14 Clients Who Lack Decision-Making Capacity

When social workers act on behalf of clients who lack the capacity to make informed decisions, social workers should take reasonable steps to safeguard the interests and rights of those clients.

1.15 Interruption of Services

Social workers should make reasonable efforts to ensure continuity of services in the event that services are interrupted by factors such as unavailability, relocation, illness, disability, or death.

1.16 Termination of Services

(a) Social workers should terminate services to clients and professional relationships with them when such services and relationships are no longer required or no longer serve the clients' needs or interests.

(b) Social workers should take reasonable steps to avoid abandoning clients who are still in need of services. Social workers should withdraw services precipitously only under unusual circumstances, giving careful consideration to all factors in the situation and taking care to minimize possible adverse effects. Social workers should assist in making appropriate arrangements for continuation of services when necessary.

(c) Social workers in fee-for-service settings may terminate services to clients who are not paying an overdue balance if the financial contractual arrangements have been made clear to the client, if the client does not pose an imminent danger to self or others, and if the clinical and other consequences of the current nonpayment have been addressed and discussed with the client.

(d) Social workers should not terminate services to pursue a social, financial, or sexual relationship with a client.

(e) Social workers who anticipate the termination or interruption of services to clients should notify clients promptly and seek the transfer, referral, or continuation of services in relation to the clients' needs and preferences.

(f) Social workers who are leaving an employment setting should inform clients of appropriate options for the continuation of services and of the benefits and risks of the options. (NASW, 1996:7-15)

Values and Ethics Considerations in Health Care Settings

The following client-related social work values, principles, and ethical standards have particular significance in health care settings.

The Value of the Dignity and Worth of the Person

The dignity and worth of the person takes on special significance in health care settings where we sometimes work with persons who are severely deteriorated, deformed, demented, deranged, or dying.

In addition, the client population of health care settings sometimes resembles a *microcosm* (a small replica) of society, in that it may include rich and poor, young and old, "saints and sinners," geniuses and mentally retarded persons, people of a variety of races, subcultures, religions, both males and females—some of whom are heterosexual and some homosexual—corporation heads, laborers, rock stars, athletes, and politicians.

As professional social workers, we are challenged to remember that every individual is of value. We accept each "person" regardless of his or her behavior. Each has a right to fulfill his or her potential. We individualize people and address our approach and services to *their* needs. We reach out to vulnerable people and advocate for them, and we avoid imposing our values and norms on them, but instead seek out and respect theirs and work within the framework of who *they* are.

The Ethical Standard of Client Confidentiality

The word *confidentiality* literally means "with faith" or "with trust." In health care settings, clients are highly vulnerable. Not only will you see them in their bedclothes or even naked, but they are "stripped of their customary supports" (Goffman, 1961) when in institutional settings such as hospitals and nursing homes. This vulnerability can cause clients to share things about themselves they might not ordinarily discuss, which later can add to their feelings of vulnerability. In addition, you will have access to their medical records, which often detail much personal information. Finally, you may encounter someone you know, or know of, among clients and their families—whether a former lover, a member of the clergy, a former teacher, or some public figure.

It is essential that you keep what you know about clients to yourself. Never "gossip," even to your family, friends, or colleagues. Record only what you would be willing for them to read, and keep confidential files locked.

Trust is the *sine qua non* (prerequisite) of effective social work practice. Violation of this trust will tend to diminish your credibility as a professional in the eyes of anyone who witnesses it.

Exceptions to the confidentiality standard include cases of public health dangers, threatened suicide or homicide, or other criminal behavior. In these instances, social workers simply inform clients that they cannot promise confidentiality.

The Ethical Standard of Client Self-Determination

Health care settings often pose important questions for patients and their families that cover a wide range of topics, such as the following:

- Whether to initiate or continue life support equipment
- Whether to have the recommended medical or surgical procedure
- Whether to accept the treatment that will reduce the symptoms or even extend life, but cause unpleasant side effects
- Which treatment option to select
- Whether to tell *significant others* (special people) about their health condition
- What to do about their lives in the future
- Whether to go to a nursing home or home after discharge from the hospital

In addition, the self-determination standard takes on special significance in health care settings because there is some evidence that when people experience a strong sense of loss of control over their lives, they tend to "give up the struggle," which can negatively affect their recovery (Schmale, 1972; Seligman, 1975; Levy, 1974).

Thus, it is very important for the social worker to (1) assist the client and/or family to gain access to needed information on which to base *informed decisions*; (2) assist them in identifying and assessing their options to make an appropriate selection; and (3) support their preferences and assist them in realizing them.

The Value of Social Justice

It is our obligation to support and actively promote equal opportunity and equitable treatment for all people—regardless of our personal feelings about them, their health condition, or their behavior. In spite of our own views about politics, morality, religion, and so forth, as professionals, we come to realize that social justice must exist for everyone or it may not exist for anyone.

Values and Ethics Conflicts

From time to time, practice situations arise that cause professionals some sense of uncertainty, strain, or temptation concerning their professional values and ethics. These are known as *values and ethics conflicts*. Such conflicts tend to be related to (1) client health conditions, personal characteristics, or behavior; (2) organizational situations or practices; or (3) community resource provider promotional efforts.

Client-Related Conflicts

Values and ethics conflicts in health settings can be stimulated by subjective reactions of social workers to clients' health conditions or their behavior. Such conflicts can impair social workers' ability to uphold their professional values and ethics, as depicted in the following examples:

- The patient's health condition is so deteriorated or impaired that you may privately question whether he or she is worth the costly care being supplied.

- The patient has a health problem that arouses emotion-laden memories of some family situation of your own.
- The patient has personal characteristics that are so like your own that you experience considerable distress that "this could be you."
- The patient has health problems that are the result of behaviors such as physical or sexual abuse, drug or alcohol dependency, homosexuality, or induced abortion, about which you may have some value-laden feelings.
- The patient is determined to go home following release, or the family is determined to take him or her home, when you strongly believe that even with all available resources, the patient will be unable to manage the needed care for his or her health condition.

Organization-Related Conflicts

Values and ethics conflicts may also arise from situations involving the organizational setting itself, as in the following examples:

- An administrator in the setting asks you to talk with members of the patient's family, who have been complaining a lot about the patient's care, in order to "get them off our backs."
- An administrator in the setting asks you to lead a series of group meetings for family members of recently admitted patients, using a manual prepared by the corporation headquarters that does not provide for the relatives to freely talk about their feelings and concerns, but rather is designed to persuade them to "disengage" from monitoring their loved one's care and simply entrust the care to the facility.
- It is evident that the health care facility is seriously understaffed, and numerous incidents of patient neglect and overuse of physical and chemical restraints have occurred.
- When you have tried to identify and reach out to patients who are "at risk," you sometimes find that their private physicians resent what they see as interference with "their patient."
- "Patient rights," outlined in writing by the organization, are sometimes violated.

- The for-profit organization appears to be basing its decisions regarding intake and discharge more on the adequacy of the insurance coverage than on the person's need for treatment.
- The physician insists that you are to arrange for the patient's discharge before you think it is possible to do so without compromising the client's or family's well-being.
- One or more patients complain to you that another professional in the setting has been physically, emotionally, or sexually abusive to them.

Community Liaison-Related Conflicts

Values and ethics conflicts also can arise in the course of linking clients with community resources. In their role as *brokers* (people who know the resource options and help clients to link up with the one best suited to their needs), social workers are in a position of vulnerability to influence by personal considerations in their community resource preferences. This has become especially true in recent years as for-profit organizations have proliferated in the health sector of the economy, often creating a "tight marketplace." Examples include community mental health centers, nursing homes, home care agencies, and medical equipment suppliers.

As a result of this increase in business-oriented service suppliers, social workers in health care settings may become the target of a sometimes bewildering bombardment of promotional materials, gifts, invitations to expensive lunches, and offers of special favors, all designed to induce social workers to steer clients to their service. There is probably nothing inherently wrong with social workers accepting these things, as long as it does not interfere with ongoing objective assessment of the comparative quality of clients' available resource options.

Coping with Values and Ethics Conflicts

There is no easy answer for dealing with these types of conflicts that social workers sometimes face in their practice in health care settings. In coping with those conflicts which are stimulated by subjective responses to *client* characteristics, social workers simply need to recall the admonition to "keep personal needs and feelings separate from the professional relationship." To deal with those conflicts raised by situations involving the *organizational setting*, social workers may be aided by remembering to "keep your commitments to your employing organization" but also respect "the primacy of the client's interests and well-being." Finally, when faced with conflicts that arise from promotional efforts of some business-oriented *community resource agency*, it is best to remember that "professional behavior should be characterized by honesty and integrity."

As social workers mature in their professionalism, they generally realize that the values and ethics of their profession can help them resolve the temptations that inevitably arise. It is the nurturance of professional knowledge, blended with and tempered by professional values and ethics, that cultivates social worker skills, which are addressed in the next section.

SKILL REQUIREMENTS

The Meaning of Skill

In everyday life, we think of skill as the ability to do something well, whether riding a bike, laying bricks, or performing brain surgery.

One thing that distinguishes the skill of a professional from that of a bike rider or bricklayer is the level of knowledge required to perform the activity well. The level of required knowledge reflects the level of *complexity* and *stability* of the phenomenon involved. Complexity refers to the multiplicity of factors. Level of stability involves the extent to which these factors are constant or changing, that is, dynamic. In other words, if every human being and human problem were identical and singular, and every client responded the same during the helping process, social work practice would be more like laying bricks.

Another distinguishing characteristic of professional skill is that it is constrained by professional values and ethics. That is, there are things we *could* but would not do because we believe them to be a violation of what our profession upholds as important and worthwhile or appropriate behavior.

Thus, *professional skill* is not "mechanical," but involves the ability to act appropriately by drawing upon a body of knowledge and a set of values and ethics while one is interacting with a complex set of often-changing conditions. Likewise, professional social work skills are not learned simply by observing others performing them, nor only from practicing them, but are rooted in (1) knowledge of human behavior and the social environment, social welfare policy and programs, methods of social work practice, and research and evaluation methods and in (2) the values and ethics of social work.

Four Characteristics of Professional Skill

As a result of this relationship between practice activity and the knowledge, values, and ethics of one's profession, the practice activity of a professional is expected to exhibit the following characteristics:

1. *Conscious*—performed with awareness of what you are doing
2. *Purposeful*—performed with an objective of what you are trying to achieve
3. *Disciplined*—performed, not impulsively, but with control
4. *Responsible*—performed with mindfulness of your obligations to the values and ethics of the profession

The Meaning of Social Work Skills

Thus, we can define *social work skills* as the application of social work knowledge, values, and ethics to the performance of social work practice activity.

Actually, any or all activities of social workers in the course of their practice, whether in direct services to clients, consultation, community liaison work, policy/program planning and development, teaching, or research and evaluation, are "skills," that is, skilled activities, if they are rooted in social work knowledge, values, and ethics and, as a result, are conscious, purposeful, disciplined, and responsible.

Generic Social Work Skills

Generic social work skills are those which are common to all social work practice and which largely revolve around direct services to clients. There are various approaches to categorizing social work skills. The way we categorize them reflects the basic steps and associated activities in the helping process of social work (DiNitto and McNeece, 1997:71-73; Morales and Sheafor, 1989:249).

Skilled Activities in Helping	Stages of Helping Process
1. Engagement	Engagement
2. Observation	Data Collection
3. Assessment	Assessment
4. Cooperative planning	Contracted intervention planning
5. Intervention modality	Plan implementation
6. Research/evaluation	Evaluation of progress/effect
7. Termination/closure	Termination
8. Communication	(Throughout the helping process)
9. Empathy	(Throughout the helping process)

In addition to these skills associated with the helping process, basic social work education helps develop a broad range of research skills as well as skills that are specific to group and community intervention.

The Difference Between Skills and Techniques

A skill is broader than a technique. A skill is a category of performance ability that identifies *what* you are doing, whereas a technique is a specific behavior or set of behaviors used in skill performance that identifies *how* you are doing it. For example, "active listening" is a communication skills technique. For each of the previous skill areas, or categories of performance ability, there is a set of associated techniques or behaviors used in skill performance (Morales and Sheafor, 1989:246, 248).

Special Skills Required in Social Work in the Health Field

Earlier, we discussed the special knowledge areas required for social work in health care settings. The special skills for social work practice in health care settings are associated with those special knowledge areas: (1) the client population and problem area; (2) the organizational setting; (3) the community characteristics and resources; (4) the specific intervention modalities; and (5) the methods of research, program evaluation, and documentation appropriate to the particular setting. Delineation of these relationships follows.

Client Population and Problem Area

Knowledge of the client population and problem area served by the health care setting, such as (1) the usual path, treatment, or management of the disorder(s), (2) the role of biological, psychological, and sociocultural variables in the onset, course, and effects of the disorder(s), and (3) the role of human diversity variables in patient and family behavior concerning health care, illness responses, and the sick role, will enhance the social worker's skill in the following practice activities:

1. Engagement, observation, assessment, cooperative planning, intervention, evaluation, termination, and overall communication and empathy associated with the process of helping patients and their families
2. Communicating with members of other health professions in the setting (because you "speak their language" and they are impressed with your insight and sensitivity to the client population and problem area)

Organizational Setting

Knowledge of the characteristics of the organizational setting (such as whether it is for profit or nonprofit, secular or sectarian, its mission and function(s), the level of health service intervention, authority structure, types of health professions and occupations in the setting and their roles and role expectations of social work, the organizational policy, rules, and regulations, in addition to interdisciplinary teamwork principles and problems) will enable the social worker to develop skill in the following practice activities:

1. Developing the social worker role in the organizational system so that it becomes a valued, complementary, integrated, and

efficient component of that system, one that is well adapted to organizational constraints, priorities, and expectations
2. Facilitating interdisciplinary teamwork
3. Informal client advocacy with other staff in the setting

Community Characteristics and Resources

Knowledge of the characteristics, resources, and resource needs of the particular community will likely enhance the social worker's skill in these practice activities:

1. Interagency communication
2. Linking clients to resources
3. Community program/policy planning and development
4. Liaison work between the practice setting and community

Specific Intervention Modalities

Social worker knowledge of intervention methods/approaches that are particularly well-suited to the needs of the particular client population, problem area, and organization will enable the social worker to develop skill in effectively helping clients to resolve their problems.

Research, Program Evaluation, and Documentation Needs

Social worker knowledge of methods of research, program evaluation, and documentation that are appropriate to and/or required by the organization setting and its funding sources will serve the social worker well in developing skill in the following areas:

1. Designing and conducting research that will help develop the practice knowledge base of social work in health care
2. Evaluating the effectiveness of the social work program in the setting as a basis for further development of that program
3. Documenting what is required for maximizing funding reimbursement to the setting
4. Encouraging interprofessional coordination by documenting case activity in medical records to inform other professional staff of it

In the next section, we will explore some dimensions of service interventions in social work in health care settings.

DIMENSIONS OF HELPING

The Mission of Social Work

Preamble

The primary mission of the social work profession is to enhance human well-being and help meet the basic human needs of all people, with particular attention to the needs and empowerment of people who are vulnerable, oppressed, and living in poverty. A historic and defining feature of social work is the profession's focus on individual well-being in a social context and the well-being of society. Fundamental to social work is attention to the environmental forces that create, contribute to, and address problems in living.

Social workers promote social justice and social change with and on behalf of clients. "Clients" is used inclusively to refer to individuals, families, groups, organizations, and communities. Social workers are sentitive to cultural and ethnic diversity and strive to end discrimination, oppression, poverty, and other forms of social injustice. These activities may be in the form of direct practice, community organizing, supervision, consultation, adminstration, advocacy, social and political action, policy development and implementation, education, and research and evaluation. Social workers seek to enhance the capacity of people to address their own needs. Social workers also seek to promote the responsiveness of organizations, communities, and other social institutions to individuals' needs and social problems.

The mission of the social work profession is rooted in a set of core values. These core values, embraced by social workers throughout the profession's history, are the foundation of social work's unique purpose and perspective:

• Service
• Social justice
• Dignity and worth of the person

- Importance of human relationships
- Integrity
- Competence

This constellation of core values reflects what is unique to the social work profession. Core values, and the principles that flow from them, must be balanced within the context and complexity of the human experience. (NASW, 1996:1)

Toward this end, professional social workers *serve* clients, through direct or indirect interventions, with the goal of restoring or enhancing their social functioning, that is, person-in-environment fit.

Direct and Indirect Social Work Services in Health Care

The basic social worker functions in health settings (NASW, 1987) identify areas of service activity and can be grouped by *direct* services, provided directly to or for the client, and *indirect* services, which are performed on behalf of or to benefit some population of potential clients.

Direct service functions include

- case finding and outreach,
- assessment of need for social work services,
- intervention planning,
- intervention (treatment),
- preadmission planning,
- discharge planning,
- information and referral,
- advocacy for a client,
- protection of rights or entitlement of a client,
- health promotion and maintenance,
- preventive, remedial, and rehabilitative measures, and
- provision of continuity of care—including guaranteed access and effective utilization.

Indirect service functions include

- advocacy for a population,
- consultation,

- liaison with the community,
- policy and program planning and development,
- quality assurance,
- research,
- social work field instruction, and
- teaching (other than field instruction).

Social Worker Roles

Roles are labels for actors that identify the function or "part" they are performing. Depending on which function a social worker is performing at any given time, his or her role in intervention may include that of

- an advocate who fights for or defends client rights;
- a broker who knows all the relevant resources and links the client with the most appropriate ones;
- a case manager who assesses a client's needs, links that client with needed resources, and coordinates and oversees resource delivery;
- a consultant who provides expert opinions to others, when asked;
- a counselor who engages in personalized interpersonal interaction with a client, which involves the client's feelings, attitudes, perceptions, or behaviors;
- a liaison who acts as a "go-between," link, or bridge between two or more people or organizations;
- a mediator who facilitates conflict resolution between parties;
- a researcher who develops new knowledge;
- a planner who prepares a design for a course of action; and/or
- a teacher who transmits knowledge to others.

The Social Work Helping Process

The social work profession conceives of a particular helping process, or series of steps or stages, in service intervention with clients. This conceptualized process serves to remind practitioners that professional social work intervention is disciplined and orderly;

it requires client involvement, systematic gathering and interpretation of relevant information, and planning with the client before "intervention" itself is initiated, followed by ongoing monitoring and final evaluation of the intervention progress, effectiveness, and outcome, and ultimately concludes with "closure" or termination of the intervention process. This sequential process includes the following states (DeNitto and McNeece, 1997:71-73):

1. Engagement of the client
2. Data collection
3. Assessment/interpretation of the data
4. Cooperative intervention planning
5. Intervention
6. Monitoring and final evaluation of progress and outcome
7. Termination of service

The Meaning of Intervention

This helping process is the conceptualized series of steps that precedes, includes, and follows the intervention itself. Theoretically, the intervention, or what is sometimes called the "treatment" or "treatment modality," is what is actually done in an effort to address the client's problem(s). Practically, it is difficult to separate the steps that precede and follow the intervention from the intervention itself because all social worker interaction with the client throughout the process has therapeutic potential.

Four Client Levels of Intervention

The "client" of social work services, or interventions, in the health field may be an individual patient (one on one), all or part of a patient's family, any other small group of people, or another larger sector of the community or society—such as the people in a neighborhood, a population of people concerned with a particular health problem, all residents of a treatment center, rehabilitation center, or halfway house, or all patients in a day treatment, day care, or other outpatient program. The "client" is the person or group that requests and/or will benefit from the social work intervention.

Intervention Objectives

Although the overall goal of social work is to restore or enhance the social functioning of clients, the more immediate *objective* of intervention may be to

- modify attitudes, perceptions, feelings, or behaviors;
- improve interpersonal relationships or communication;
- facilitate decision making and self-determination;
- enhance adaptation and coping capacity; and
- sustain or enhance mental or physical comfort and functioning.

Intervention Approaches

In addressing such objectives, a variety of approaches may be considered, the selection of which depends on assessment of the client's needs and capacities. Essentially, there are a relatively small number of such approaches:

1. Counseling in some form
2. Education or skill training
3. Resource information and resource linkage assistance
4. Advocacy to help the client obtain what he or she needs and is entitled to have
5. Modification of the environment to adapt it to client needs
6. Community resource development

Affective-Expressive and Concrete-Instrumental Interventions

Historically, social workers have tended to categorize their interventions in health care settings as either (1) affective-expressive or (2) concrete-instrumental ones.

Affective-expressive interventions are thought of as the various forms of "counseling," which involve a process of personalized interpersonal interaction between the social worker and client in which the focus is on attitudes, feelings, perceptions, decisions, or behaviors of the client. Frequently, such services target client problems that are related to *adjustment* to the health service or facility or to the diagnosis, prognosis, or medical treatment plan. However, in mental health settings, affective-expressive interventions are also often directed toward treating the health problem itself. Such interventions are termed "affective-expressive" because they focus on "affect," that is, feelings/moods, and "expression," or behavior.

Concrete-instrumental interventions, on the other hand, are thought of as those which revolve around resource information and referral activity, that is, linking the client with needed resources—such as assisting with arrangements for admission and aftercare, the care of the patient's family during his or her absence or disability, assistance with transportation to health services, helping to obtain medical aids and appliances, or assisting with financial arrangements for the patient's care.

In other words, concrete-instrumental interventions tend to be thought of as tangible services in which the social worker acts as an "agent" for the client; they focus on social environmental problems, needs, and resources and often are associated with patient problems relating to admission and aftercare.

More recently, however, social workers are realizing that this traditional distinction between affective-expressive and concrete-instrumental social work interventions is somewhat artificial (Blazyk and Canavan, 1985). This is because preadmission and discharge planning often need to involve the attitudes, feelings, perceptions, decisions, or behaviors of patients and/or their family members; conversely, patients with problems of adjustment to the health care service or facility or to the diagnosis, prognosis, or treatment plan, or patients whose primary health problem is a mental rather than a physical one, often have a variety of concrete concerns and needs.

The Concept of Psychosocial Problems

"Psychosocial problems" are problems with both psychological and social environmental components, which reflect the inevitable influence each arena has on the other.

Fundamental to social work in health care is the perspective that the social functioning of people reflects what is variously termed the interaction, intersection, interface, or transactions between the "person" with attitudes, feelings, perceptions, and behavior patterns and his or her "environment," with its presenting situation, resources, and supports (Germain and Gitterman, 1980).

Thus, a person's social functioning reflects both his or her interpretation of a situation and the actual situation. For this reason, the interventions of the social worker address "psychosocial" problems that impair optimal social functioning.

Intervention Methods

Intervention methods, sometimes called treatment modalities, are more or less specific techniques or models for intervention, each with a premise concerning how or why it ought to help solve the problem.

There are many intervention or "treatment" approaches that the social worker may view as a repertoire of options, the choice of which depends on the nature of the client's problem, needs, and capacities. In one text (Kerson, 1989), the combined social workers who contributed case studies to that anthology of readings identify more than twenty such treatment modalities or types of interventions that they have used in their practice in health care settings: crisis intervention, problem solving, education and information, task-oriented counseling, ego-oriented casework, confrontation, peer group therapy, assertiveness training, group work, case management, family therapy, behavior modification, entitlement and advocacy, concrete services, milieu therapy, skill training, psychoanalysis, cognitive therapy, relaxation therapy, modeling, supportive counseling, reminiscence therapy, and nondirective client-centered counseling.

Premises of Alternate Interventions

The uses of these interventions for various client needs in the health field suggest the following premises of their selection:

People may benefit from:

- *education and information* to make informed decisions and take charge of their lives and health;
- outreach coupled with caring *confrontation* to get them to address their health behavior or health problem;

- rehearsing those behaviors which are required to change a problem situation (*task-oriented counseling*);
- social interaction (discussion, recreational activity, shared task activity, etc.) with a group of other people they respect and can identify with in order to change their attitudes, feelings, perceptions, or behaviors (*group therapy/peer group therapy*);
- learning new skills in order to change problem situations or develop adaptive behaviors (*skill training*);
- direct, focused, practical, supportive assistance when in a "crisis" (*crisis intervention*);
- learning *problem-solving skills,* such as partializing and focusing;
- learning to interpret events as less threatening and to recognize positive rather than self-defeating messages (*cognitive therapy*);
- a supportive environment or "milieu" (*milieu therapy*);
- counseling with their family groups to identify and eliminate dysfunctional patterns of communication within them (*family therapy*);
- ego-building to cope with stress (*ego-oriented casework*);
- developing insight into past experience to help cope with the present (*psychoanalysis*);
- having a professional who is designated to coordinate service delivery when they require services from a variety of agencies or specialists (*case management*);
- positive reinforcement of progress in their efforts to make behavioral changes (*behavior modification*);
- having someone to "fight for" their rights for them (*advocacy*);
- *concrete services* and resources to meet basic material needs instead of, or before, services to address emotional or behavioral problems;
- learning how to assert one's position on issues without attacking or provoking others (*assertiveness training*);
- learning how to induce a period of relaxation to avert unhealthy behavioral responses (*relaxation therapy*);
- observing other people demonstrate appropriate behaviors in order to learn them (*modeling*);

- recollecting and reminiscing about "good times" in the past to help restore their sense of ego integrity when they are overwhelmed by life change events (*reminiscence therapy*); and
- having someone listen and provide *support* while they think through their problems and restore their ego functioning (*supportive counseling*).

The Meaning of Counseling in Social Work

With the exception of education and information, milieu therapy, problem solving, skill training, case management, advocacy, and concrete services, the treatment modalities or interventions identified in the Kerson (1989) text fall under the category of "counseling."

Counseling is a broad term that refers to a personalized interpersonal process of helping that relies heavily on verbal and nonverbal communication between the social worker and client(s). Counseling may be provided to an individual, family, or other small group.

Counseling in social work is generally thought of as the medium through which social workers attempt to "treat" problems in social functioning that require a focus on attitudes, feelings, perceptions, or behaviors of the *person*. Because counseling involves emotional and behavioral functioning, it is sometimes called an "affective-expressive" activity.

The objective of counseling may be to

1. change a person's attitudes, feelings, perceptions, or behaviors;
2. change interpersonal relationships and communication patterns;
3. help the client to think through and make some needed decisions; and/or
4. sustain or enhance a person's coping capacity.

While counseling can, and often does, include teaching new skills, providing needed information or education, advocacy, or linking clients with needed concrete resources, such activities must be coupled with a personalized interpersonal process and linked with one or more of the previous four objectives to be considered "counseling."

Social work is distinguished from other helping professions by its dual focus on the *person and the environment*. Therefore, if social workers who do counseling wish to retain their identity as social workers, they need to sustain this dual focus. In theory, social workers who disregard the social environmental context of the client as a person and address only the client's intrapsychic functioning are not practicing social work.

The Theoretical Perspective of Care or Caring

Once emerged, few of the major mental or physical health problems today are amenable to complete "cure." Earlier in this century when social work in health care began, the major health problems in the United States were acute *infectious* diseases (those which are caused by bacteria or viruses), such as typhoid, typhus, pneumonia, tuberculosis, and other bacterial infections. As a result of their prevalence, life expectancy was about 60 percent of what it is today. However, as public health measures and medical technology developed, these diseases were brought under control and more people began to live longer.

One result of longer life expectancy is that *chronic* health problems (permanent and incurable ones) have now emerged as the major health problems. This is because chronic disorders, such as heart disease, hypertension, cancer, type II diabetes, strokes, and arthritis, tend to emerge with advancing age. In addition, younger people with chronic diseases and disabilities, such as epilepsy, type I diabetes, severe mental illness, mental retardation and other developmental disabilities, also live longer now because of the development of anticonvulsive drugs, insulin, and antipsychotic drugs, as well as antibiotics that help control the infectious diseases that once tended to shorten people's lives.

Although heart disease, hypertension, strokes, and cancer are the major causes of death and disability, certain psychosocial problems are also gaining prominence, sometimes as contributing causes of chronic disease. Examples of such *psychosocial problems* include alcoholism and other drug abuse, cigarette smoking, eating disorders, domestic violence, rape and other forms of sexual abuse, homicide, suicide, and motor vehicle accidents.

Neither the chronic health problems nor the psychosocial or behavioral ones are "curable" in the same sense that infectious diseases often are. For this reason, the focus must be on *care interventions* (supportive forms of assistance) to help prevent health problems, to enhance what recovery is possible once health problems have emerged, and to help compensate for the impairments associated with chronic or terminal problems once they reach that stage:

> Since most serious diseases and disabilities are likely to prove relatively intractable if they cannot be prevented, the role of therapeutic medicine should be modified to include as the major commitment the concept of care. Such a change would carry major implications for medical science and service and should affect the content and orientation of medical education. (McLachlan and McKeown, 1971:48)

Since the terms "care" and "caring" are so commonly but variously used, it is important to clarify what they mean. I agree with David Mechanic, who wrote:

> It is unfortunately common for many physicians to conceive of the caring functions of medical care as simply the expression of kindness and acceptance of the patient. While this is no trivial aspect, *caring constitutes* a much wider *range of techniques based* not only on human feeling, or even on the techniques usually associated with psychotherapy, but *on scientific knowledge of how to provide human support. . . . In short, caring is a technology, the dimensions of which can be concretely identified, studied, manipulated and transmitted to practitioners who apply the technology in concrete situations.* Caring is thus much more than a communication of feeling. . . . (emphasis added) (1978:309)

The Purpose of Caring

Oftentimes, people need extensive supportive types of assistance to

1. help prevent the onset of health problems;
2. enhance the "cure" process and keep health and other human problems from compounding or developing into a worsened state once emerged; and

3. maximize comfort and function once health problems have become chronic and/or terminal.

"Health" is a state of biological, psychological, and social well-being, not simply the absence of disease (WHO, 1978). Care interventions, or supportive kinds of assistance, are directed toward a combination of biological (physical), psychological (mental and emotional), and social well-being. For this reason, caring is an interdisciplinary and biopsychosocial approach to helping.

An underlying premise of the care approach to helping is that service providers must "cooperate with," not do things to, the patient and family to

1. engage them in efforts to achieve the goal appropriate to the patient's health status level (prevention, repair, compensation), and
2. promote their self-determination and sense of control and mastery needed to ward off feelings of helplessness, powerlessness, and "giving up."

The Rationale for Care Interventions

The *rationale* for providing supportive assistance, that is, care interventions, at all three levels of health service intervention is as follows:

1. At the *primary level,* initially, some health problems emerge, in part, because of one or more of the following:
   a. People engage in self-destructive or high-risk behavior.
   b. People are exposed to environmental dangers.
   c. People experience stressful life change events that reduce their coping level and resistance to health problems.
2. At the *secondary level,* when people are ill or injured with acute episodes of health problems that could be cured, repaired, or whose development could be slowed or stopped, the following problems arise:
   a. People do not always recognize that they are ill or injured or need help.
   b. People do not always know where to go to seek appropriate help.

   c. People sometimes are afraid of seeking such help.

   d. People sometimes feel they cannot "afford" to accept the help, for financial reasons or due to other responsibilities.

   e. People sometimes have other barriers to getting the needed help, for example, transportation, discrimination, or cultural beliefs.

   f. People with acute health conditions, once they gain access to the needed treatment service, often experience impairment of their functional capacity and/or comfort, which, if not supported for them, can act as a barrier to attaining their level of potential recovery.

   g. People who are ready for release but still need some special care are more likely to relapse if supportive assistance is not provided to help ensure continuity of care.

3. At the *tertiary level,* when people have chronic and/or terminal health conditions that cannot be "cured"; the following issues must be considered:

   a. People often experience considerable impairment of comfort and functioning, whether mental, physical, or social.

   b. People require extensive supportive forms of assistance to help them compensate for such impairment (Morris and Anderson, 1975).

Interpersonal Supports

"Interpersonal supports" are interactions and communications and relationships with other people that are experienced as emotionally supportive, that is, as indications to patients that someone cares about them. Examples might include reaching-out to people in need, calling them by the name they prefer, respecting their cultural and other human diversity characteristics, showing interest in and attending to their thoughts and feelings, being available when needed, showing prompt attention and responsiveness to their needs, encouraging their ability to make their own decisions and do for themselves when able, facilitating their having and doing what they find enjoyable, being accepting of them as individuals, and assisting them to obtain what they need and are willing to receive.

In fact, the theoretical perspective I call "caring" is rooted in the principle that the supportive interventions required for health main-

tenance, repair, and compensation *must* include interpersonal interactions, communications, and relationships that are experienced by
the client as "feeling cared about"—since the belief that one is of
value is the source of personal motivation and empowerment,
which is the sine qua non of health maintenance, recovery, and
coping with chronic health problems.

Limitations of Social Work Intervention in Health Care Settings

Social work intervention in health care settings is often constrained by a variety of conditions, usually relating to the client,
setting, or community.

Client-Related Constraints

In both mental and physical health settings, the patients themselves are sometimes unable to participate fully in any type of social
work intervention, either because they are children or because they
are too ill or handicapped to communicate, express preferences,
make decisions, or provide needed information.

As a result, the social worker may need to work with family
members, a legal guardian, or others with legal authority to act on
the client's behalf, such as one with "power of attorney." In lieu of
the availability of such a person, the social worker may be required
to initiate the legal process to appoint a guardian for the client.

Organization-Related Constraints

Depending on the characteristics of the organizational setting of
practice, there may be constraints on social work intervention in
terms of the following: (1) available time to work with clients when
they are not engaged in other program activities or before they are
discharged; (2) which kinds of services are reimbursable; (3) which
kinds of services are acceptable to organizational policy (for example, Catholic organizations are unlikely to allow social worker interventions that facilitate access to abortion or "artificial" methods of
contraception); and (4) which staff members of the organization are
allocated responsibility for which types of services. For example, in

some health settings, persons other than social workers may be assigned responsibility for preadmission and/or discharge planning or counseling. In addition, oftentimes, an interdisciplinary team of health professionals, rather than an individual, jointly decides upon appropriate interventions.

Community-Related Constraints

Finally, the options for social work intervention are sometimes limited by community-related conditions. For example, you may find that the community simply does not have certain resources that you feel the client needs, in which case the social worker needs to be as "creative" as possible to find alternate solutions. These may include seeking private or little-known benefactors to purchase something, or they may require the social worker to help develop a resource, such as a support group; it may also be helpful to consult with a professional who has expertise in that resource area (such as a particular type of medical equipment) regarding possible substitutes for the recommended one.

Another common situation is that the patient may not be from the local community or is being released to a facility or family member in some other, often distant community. In these cases, considerable exploration is usually required to determine what the resources are in that other community.

A common, and particularly challenging, community-related situation for social workers occurs when the patient is being released to a very rural and remote area in another state where community resources are practically nonexistent. In such situations, it can be productive to telephone one or more large agencies in your own community that provide that type of service to ask if they know the location and phone number of a comparable service in the urban area closest to where the patient is going. By making contact with the latter organizations, the social worker can often gain considerable assistance in working out a plan for continuity of the patient's care, including access to the available local resources.

SUMMARY

At the base of every profession is the claim that it has a special body of knowledge that enables its members to understand and address the phenomena encompassed by their arena of practice.

All social work practice requires knowledge of (1) human behavior and the social environment, (2) social welfare policy and programs, (3) social work practice, and (4) social work research methods. Only social work practice knowledge is unique to the social work profession and must be continually developed through ongoing research within the profession.

In addition, social work practice in a health care setting requires some specialized knowledge of (1) the client population and problem area, (2) the particular organizational setting, (3) the community and its resources, (4) specific intervention modalities, and (5) research, evaluation, and documentation suited to the setting.

Besides having a body of knowledge, a profession must have a set of values and ethics to guide members' practice of that profession. The new Code of Ethics of the NASW lays out some core values, principles, and standards of the social work profession that are of special relevance to practice in health care. Challenges that sometimes confront social workers concerning their professional values and ethics often arise in relation to client, organizational, or community liaison situations. However, the resolution of such conflicts is also often aided by reviewing and reflecting on this Code of Ethics.

Social worker skills for practice in health care settings are cultivated through specialized knowledge and are both inspired and constrained by the guiding values and ethics of the profession—resulting in practice activity that is conscious, purposeful, disciplined, and responsible.

From professional knowledge comes *conscious* practice activity—knowing what you are doing. From knowledge also comes *purposeful* practice activity—knowing what your objective is, why you are doing it. From the values and ethics of the profession comes *disciplined* activity—control of impulses—as well as *responsible* behavior—activity that is mindful of social workers' obligations to

SECTION II:
SETTINGS AT THE THREE LEVELS
OF INTERVENTION

Chapter 3

Social Work
in Primary Care Settings

HISTORICAL BACKGROUND

The early work of social workers in settlement houses during the latter quarter of the nineteenth century involved engaging the community in social action efforts to modify social and physical environmental conditions seen as detrimental to public health, including those related to housing, workplaces, sewage and water, and lack of education:

> . . . their goal was to bridge the gap between the classes and races, to eliminate the sources of distress, and to improve urban living and working conditions. Like the public health reformers, with whom they frequently cooperated, theirs was the preventive approach. (Trattner, 1989:147)

In 1905, Dr. Richard C. Cabot hired social workers to work in his medical clinic at Massachusetts General Hospital. These workers were to make home visits (Oktay, 1995:1891) to bring back to the medical and nursing staff an understanding of the conditions in the patient's home, work, and community that were relevant to the patient's health problem (Cabot, 1955:28); they also were to address those conditions whenever possible (Cannon, 1923:15, 30).

Social work in primary health care developed further during the Great Depression when the Social Security Act was passed in 1935, which called for social workers to be employed in the Maternal and Child Health Program and the Crippled Children's Program (Oktay, 1995).

Before World War II, most Americans obtained their medical care services through their family physician, mostly "general practitioners" and some internists and pediatricians. However, it was not until the 1960s that medical specialization was sufficiently widespread that concern began to emerge about the decline in what was termed "primary care." This marked the beginning of multiple subsequent efforts by the U.S. government to promote a return to primary care, efforts that continue today (Donaldson et al., 1996:19-20).

Beginning in the 1960s, the federal government funded such primary health care settings as migrant health centers, neighborhood health centers, and homeless health care programs, staffed by physicians who were repaying their loans under the National Health Services Act (Oktay, 1995).

Also during the 1960s, social workers were written into these federally funded neighborhood health centers as part of the Antipoverty Program and included as mandated staff in the first federally funded HMOs. Social workers have been widely used in hospital outpatient clinics, as the DRG system has reduced inpatient care and hospitals have sought alternative forms of service opportunities (Oktay, 1995:1891).

In the late 1980s, the U.S. Department of Health and Human Services (DHHS), Division of Maternal and Child Health, began to support social worker training in public health concepts (Henk, 1989). Currently, the NASW and the Council on Social Work Education (CSWE) sponsored Institute for the Advancement of Social Work Research has been cooperating with the National Institute of Mental Health (NIMH) to support research on social work in primary health care to help prevent and provide early intervention in mental disorders (Oktay, 1995:1891).

In 1990, 547 community, migrant, and homeless health centers were serving 6 million people, or about one-fourth of the nation's medically indigent (National Association of Community Health Centers, 1993). In addition, government funds support Maternal and Child Health Block Grant programs, public health department primary care programs, such as well-baby clinics, prenatal care, immunization and screening programs, and child development programs for prevention of and early intervention in child developmental problems (Oktay, 1995:1889).

However, during the conservative backlash period of the 1980s, federal funding to train primary care physicians and to support primary care services for underserved people dropped significantly, and few health care settings in the United States now provide true primary care, although many use the term to describe their services. That is, few first-contact settings provide health service that is comprehensive, coordinated, and continuous, although HMOs may come closest to providing primary care, since they have an incentive to keep people healthy and to avoid high-cost services (Oktay, 1995:1888).

Settings of Social Work in Primary Care

Social workers in primary care may be found in hospital outpatient clinics, HMOs, neighborhood health center clinics, and group medical practices (Miller, 1987:323). In addition, social workers are firmly entrenched in many of the family practice residency training centers throughout the United States, functioning in accordance with the American Academy of Family Physicians (Hess, 1985:57; Zayas and Dyche, 1992). Other sites of social work in primary care include hospital emergency rooms, free clinics, and public health departments (Ell and Morrison, 1981:355), as well as family planning clinics (Kerson and Peachey, 1989).

According to Bloom (1995:1898), major settings of social work in "primary prevention" include public schools; workplaces (e.g., employee assistance programs, accident prevention programs); recreational settings; social agencies that provide social support and skills training and education, such as self-help groups, and social and coping skills training (e.g., family life education, parenting training, assertiveness training, caregiver support, suicide prevention, grief support); and health settings, such as HMOs with prevention-oriented services.

The idea of integrating social work services into primary care practice has long received conceptual support both from the medical and social work communities. In the Health Maintenance Organization Act of 1973, the U.S. government mandated that social work services be integrated into health maintenance organizations as an essential profession to achieve the objectives of health promotion and early intervention (Badger et al., 1997:22).

Primary Health Care Concepts

In the literature, the fields of primary medicine, public health, and preventive medicine are sometimes discussed as separate disciplines, sometimes as overlapping, and sometimes as parts of a common whole. They are presented here as parts of a conceptual whole that includes the following:

1. *Professions providing primary medical care* such as family practice, internal medicine, pediatrics, physician assistants, and nurse practitioners
2. *Settings of primary health care practice,* including the solo and group practices of any of the previous professions, outpatient clinics located in hospitals, neighborhood health centers, free-standing clinics, and HMOs
3. *The field of public health*
4. *Primary prevention*, that is, efforts to prevent the occurrence of health problems

Both public health and primary care attempt to use education and information as a means to improve health behavior and prevent disease and disability. Both provide immunizations to prevent disease; both provide primary health care checkups and screening programs to achieve early intervention in health problems.

It appears that the main difference between public health and primary care is that primary prevention is a goal of public health, which is focused on the *community* more than on the individual, which is the focus in primary care. Primary medical care programs are more likely to employ social workers to address health-related psychosocial problems on a one-to-one or group basis, whereas public health programs are more apt to advocate for changes in policy and programs through legislation that will impact entire populations. However, these differences between primary care, public health, and preventive medicine are becoming increasingly blurred.

Primary Care

Technically, the term "primary care" refers to the emphasis on the patient's first entry into the health care system. The Health Maintenance Organization Act of 1973 endorsed support for primary health care in the United States (Miller, 1987:321).

In 1978, the World Health Organization named primary health care as the key to attaining health care for all people by the year 2000 (Oktay, 1995:1887) and identified its key concepts as including the terms practical, affordable, acceptable to the community, accessible and community based, and the gateway to continuity of the health care system (WHO, 1978:25).

The 1978 Assembly of the World Health Organization on Primary Care "emphasized the promotion of health, the prevention of disease, and the integration of mental and physical health services; and advocated a holistic approach that includes the physical, mental, and social aspects of health" (Oktay, 1995:1887).

Whereas the WHO concept of primary health care encompasses public health objectives of community-based health promotion and primary prevention of disease, American medical practice tends to reserve the concept of primary health care for personal health care services, excluding public health work. According to the Institute of Medicine (IOM) Committee on the Future of Primary Care:

> Primary care is the provision of *integrated, accessible* health care services by clinicians who are *accountable* for *addressing a large majority of personal health care needs*, developing a *sustained* partnership with patients, and practicing in the context of family and community. (emphasis added) (Donaldson et al., 1996:31)

Miller (1987:321) referred to these five characteristics of primary care as coordinated, accessible, comprehensive, continuous, and accountable.

The Institute of Medicine refers to the need for partnership with patients and practice in the context of family and community, suggesting a developing recognition by the medical profession that effective primary care must be a cooperative venture rather than an authoritative one and that people are influenced by interaction with other social system levels, such as family and community. The IOM also acknowledges the limitation of primary medical care without public health:

> [Primary care] will have a limited impact on health status until or unless the determinants of public and social health are addressed. . . . The aggregate benefits in health status to be gained from increasing income or education greatly outweigh the gains from medical intervention. . . . Similarly, preventing injuries from violence, child neglect, or motor vehicle crashes and deterring the adverse effects of teenage pregnancy, substance abuse, and sexually transmitted diseases are critical to the health of the community. (Donaldson et al., 1996:71)

The IOM acknowledges that *access* is a key requirement of primary care. If people do not have financial and geographic ability to obtain primary health care when it is needed, there is no way to fulfill the objectives of prevention and early intervention, both of which are related to improved population health as well as to health care cost control. Thus, universal health insurance or some other form of universal access to primary health care is a necessity (Donaldson et al., 1996:113).

The six main attributes of high-quality primary care are described as follows:

1. Primary care is grounded in both the biomedical and social sciences.
2. Primary care acknowledges the necessity sometimes of diagnostic ambiguity, given the complexity of interacting environmental factors.
3. Primary care considers physical and mental health together.
4. Primary care intrinsically provides opportunities to promote health and prevent disease.
5. Primary health will increasingly utilize computerized information systems to facilitate quality practice in multiple ways. (Donaldson et al., 1996:80-81, 88)

Primary health care recognizes the interaction of physical, mental, emotional, and social functioning of a person. *Social function-*

ing is conceived of as dealing with the ability to perform social roles, such as being a student, parent, or worker (Donaldson et al., 1996:37-38). The primary health care provider is also viewed as a "gatekeeper" to additional services (Ibid., 39).

The five main potential values of primary health care are that it (1) provides a one-stop service; (2) aids patient and family in navigating the health care system; (3) provides continuity of care; (4) offers prevention, early intervention, and health promotion; and (5) helps to link patient, family, and community (Donaldson et al., 1996:53).

Public Health

These standards have been prepared by the Social Work Section of the American Public Health Association in collaboration with the Health Quality Standards Committee of the National Association of Social Workers. They refer to the organization of the social work components of a public health program and the practice of social work in such a program.

Definition of Public Health: A commonly used definition of public health is one formulated by C.-E.A. Winslow in 1920.

According to Winslow, "Public Health is the science and art of (1) preventing diseases, (2) prolonging life, and (3) promoting health and efficiency through organized community effort for:

(a) the sanitation of the environment
(b) the control of communicable infections
(c) the education of the individual in personal hygiene
(d) the organization of medical and nursing services for the prevention and treatment of diseases
(e) the development of social machinery to insure everyone a standard of living adequate for the maintenance of health. . .

so organizing these benefits as to enable every citizen to realize his birthright of health and longevity."[1]

---

[1] C.-E.A. Winslow, "The Untilled Field of Public health," *Modern Medicine*, Vol. 2 (March 1920): 183-191.

Earlier statements of standards of social work practice in public health referred primarily to practice in official public health agencies.[2] Since that time, public health services in the curative and rehabilitative areas have been expanded, and collaborative efforts by the public and private sectors in implementing health programs with public health goals have increased. The use of the phrase "public health programs" in this statement of standards, therefore, does not refer to a specific agency or setting but rather to the policy base of a program. A public health program may be operated by the voluntary sector, e.g., Visiting Nurse Association, as well as by the public. A public health program, such as a comprehensive program for children and youth, may be one of many administered by a health agency whose primary goal may be curative rather than preventive, e.g., a children's hospital. The phrase "public health program" may also refer to a tax-supported agency operating independently as an adjunct to the official state or local department, such as a comprehensive health center of a health systems agency. (NASW, 1987:6-7)

THEORETICAL PERSPECTIVES

In spite of the varying concepts, both primary health and public health have a perspective that is biopsychosocial, holistic, sensitive to human diversity, client empowerment oriented, and rooted in epidemiology, in the primary prevention of disease and disability, and in health promotion.

Epidemiology

Primary prevention, public health, and primary health care are based on an epidemiological perspective that seeks to trace the etiology of health problems by investigating the incidence distribution of specific health problems. Epidemiology is the study of the distribution of the occurrence of health problems using such vari-

---

[2]Committee on Professional Education of the American Public Health Association, "Educational Qualifications of Social Workers in Public Health Programs," *American Journal of Public Health*, Vol. 52 (February 1962): 317-324.

ables as geographical location, climate, and time of year—as well as age, sex, ethnicity, income, educational level, and occupation. These latter six variables are indicators of social status, and their relationship to disease, disability, and death is the subject of *social epidemiology* (Engel, 1977).

Friis and Sellers (1996:376) present what they term a "guide to psychosocial epidemiology" that serves to identify some of the major independent variables, moderator variables, and dependent variables in a theoretical model of chronic disease etiology (see Table 3.1). In epidemiology, the victim is termed the *host*, the causal factor becomes the *agent*, and the context in which the two encounter is referred to as the *environment*.

Modern epidemiology is not as linked as it once was with the medical model of disease, which traditionally conceived of each health problem as having more or less a single "cause," such as a bacterium or virus. Today, epidemiology more often recognizes a complexity of interacting "causes" (Bloom, 1995:1896).

The Biopsychosocial Model

The biopsychosocial model of health and disease is usually attributed to George Engel (1977), whose seminal article, which appeared over twenty years ago in the journal *Science*, is probably among the most renowned ever written. Primary health care is rooted in the

TABLE 3.1. The Psychosocial Epidemiology of Chronic Disease

Independent Variables	Moderator Variables	Dependent Variables
Stress	Personality factors, e.g., type A behavior	Life and job satisfaction
Status incongruity	Culture	Mental health, e.g., affective states/ depression
Person-in-environment fit	Social support	Chronic disease
Life events	Lifestyle behavior	

Source: Friis, Robert H. and Sellers, Thomas A. (1996). *Epidemiology for Public Health Practice.* Gaithersburg, MD: Aspen Publishers, 376.

belief that health status is the result of a complex interaction of biological, psychological, and social, cultural, and physical environmental factors. Consequently, good health will never result from simply seeking medical intervention from any one of an array of specialist physicians, depending on the particular health problems one has already developed. Rather, the biopsychosocial model holds that good health is the result of genetic inheritance, learned behavior, cultural influences, the quality of the physical environment, socioeconomic status, age and sex, the amount and kind of stress experienced, coping mechanisms, diet, exercise, intake of dangerous drugs, social supports, sense of empowerment, and access to medical care, especially at the primary level.

It appears that mental, physical, and social health affect one another; that is, social environmental conditions can induce a sense of helplessness and depression, which in turn may induce biochemical changes that impair the immune system and increase susceptibility to disease. In addition, such socially induced depression can increase vulnerability to accidents and injuries, whether from impaired concentration and inattentiveness or high-risk behavior in search of a sense of power. On the other hand, having a disease or disability can itself produce adverse emotions due to the real or expected impact of the physical health problem on normal social-role functioning.

It may well be that once an interaction of physical, psychological, and social function factors is set in motion, a self-perpetuating cycle ensues; that is, although originally a situation, for example, a death or divorce or job loss, produced emotional depression and a compromised immune system, which led to the emergence of a physical disease of some sort, now having the physical disease itself may induce further dysfunctional emotions and social-role impairment, and so on.

Evidence suggests that mental and physical health are related. Patients with chronic illness tend to become depressed (Hill, Kelleher, and Shumaker, 1992). Five to ten percent of patients in primary care settings have been diagnosed with major depression, and two to three times that many have symptoms of mild depression (Katon and Schulberg, 1992). In addition, depressed patients tend to use health services more (Katon, 1987). According to Davis (1996:83), at least thirteen studies have confirmed that individuals with various forms of mental illness have rates of physical illness far in excess of the expected frequency of such illness in the general population. There is widespread concern that chronically mentally ill people receive a gross lack of medical care for physical health problems (Davis, 1996).

Clare (1982) found that half of the patients with a mental health problem in a primary care setting also had some type of social problem, such as with family, housing, or employment. At the same time, we know that people exposed to prolonged stress tend to have impaired immune systems (Pert et al., 1985:820s-826s; Evans, Barer, and Marmor, 1994:13). Mechanic (1994) has made a strong case for integrating mental health care into primary medical care.

Most fascinating of all is the compilation of evidence presented by Evans, Barer, and Marmor (1994) that, worldwide, there is a demonstrable direct relationship between social status and health status. This appears to be more a reflection of an individual's sense of power, control, competency, self-esteem, resources to combat stressors, self-actualization, and general well-being *associated* with social status than of income. Social class is probably one of the most useful shorthand indicators of a person's power (Freund and McGuire, 1991:31).

There is considerable evidence that "social supports" play a major role in the mitigation of stress, although valued *sources* of social support vary across cultures and need not refer to family and friends (Corin, 1994:125). Perhaps the strongest argument for professional social workers playing a major role in health care in the future is the evidence that mediating structures, such as social supports, are *the most powerful determinant of health*, and the key role of such community support in promoting a healthy society cannot be overemphasized (Kelner, 1985).

Without question, genetic inheritance plays a fundamental role in determining health status. Causes of death and length of life tend to run in families. Of course, part of the reason for this may be that younger family members tend to learn the behavior patterns of older family members—including health and illness behavior patterns, as well as work habits, mechanisms for coping with stress, and even mental attitudes toward "locus of control" (Wheaton, 1980). Although there clearly is a genetic influence, its impact can be significantly mitigated by a supportive social environment (Evans, Barer, and Marmor, 1994:20).

A Holistic Perspective

Because of the interaction of biopsychosocial factors, true primary health care requires simultaneous examination and treatment of the "whole person," including physical symptoms, emotional states, social and physical environmental conditions, cultural influences, and cognitive interpretations.

Many years ago, the World Health Organization defined health as "a physical, emotional, and social state of well-being" and not merely the "absence of disease." The WHO definition recognizes that health status is related to an individual's ability to function—physically, emotionally, and socially—and to that person's subjective sense of well-being.

Sensitivity to Human Diversity

Since social, cultural, and psychological variables are now widely recognized as playing a major role in health status by interacting with biological variables, primary health care has come to realize that variation in these variables across age, gender, ethnicity, socioeconomic class, and sexual orientation is essential information to ascertain and truly "understand"—the result of profound empathy.

This writer's conceptualization of the meaning of "sensitivity to human diversity" is as follows: (1) Knowing the other person's ethnicity, gender, age, socioeconomic class, sexual orientation, and so on, and what they mean to that person; (2) respecting the other person's human diversity characteristics; and (3) using these characteristics to adapt an approach to the other's reality, as needed, in working with the person.

There is a large body of literature on the relationships between health status and such human diversity variables as age, gender, ethnicity, and social class. This literature is central to a variety of fields, such as epidemiology, medical sociology, behavioral medicine, human development, social psychology, and medical anthropology.

It is essential that social workers in the health care field sincerely commit themselves to developing an understanding of human diversity variables as they relate to health. An excellent reference pertaining to cultural diversity for social workers and others in the helping professions is by James W. Green, who wrote, "Ethnic competence means moving beyond the job description and learning about clients through direct observation and participation in their everyday routines in naturalistic settings" (1995:97).

The Green (1995) text is interesting to read and useful in understanding how to explore with a client/patient what his or her health complaints are and what his or her understanding is of their meaning. It is clear that such an approach is vital to developing a strategy for preventive health and health promotion efforts with an individual, family, group, organization, community, or society.

Green stresses the need for social workers in health care to understand the ethnicity of their clients, while also individualizing them. He wrote, "to perceive the client's individuality as something beyond or behind, or irrelevant to these ethnographic features leaves only an insubstantial ephemera of what the individual must really be like" (1995:71-72). According to Green, in order for social workers to individualize clients within their cultural context, they must know clients' cultural resources, including the "institutions, individuals, and customs for resolving problems that are indigenous to the client's own community" (1995:95).

The meaning of a health behavior, such as drinking, smoking, diet, or physical activity, may be quite different from one culture to another. Behaviors that are unhealthy may have quite a different etiology, role, and function, and effective prevention and treatment (Green, 1995).

There is no doubt from the mounting evidence that human diversity variables are associated with *morbidity* (disease) and *mortality* (death) rates worldwide. These variables are expressed through "health behavior" and "illness behavior," which are, in turn, heavily influenced by *values and beliefs* (culture) and by an individual's sense of locus of control and *personal efficacy* (power).

Health Behavior

The individual and family must assume primary responsibility for living as much as possible in a way that encourages and promotes good health. Such "health behavior" (Cockerham, 1992:81-95) pertains to, for example, diet, exercise, abstinence from tobacco and other drugs, moderation in alcohol use, and stress management.

The challenge, of course, is to find effective ways to help people to avoid behavior that is high risk for disease or disability. It is important to avoid the pitfall of "blaming the victim," especially when commercial advertising is rampantly promoting human consumption of products that are potentially lethal. They do so by appealing to deep-seated needs, such as feeling relaxed, free, attractive, loved, and fulfilled. Sadly, much high-risk behavior may be engaged in *because* people feel "unwell" and are seeking some sort of relief.

It has been observed that people of higher socioeconomic status are more likely to engage in positive health behavior. One theory about this phenomenon is that "The sense of personal efficacy associated with higher social position encourages beliefs both in one's ability to break addictions and in the positive consequences of doing so. Beliefs in the effectiveness (or lack of it) of one's actions are both learned and reinforced by one's social position" (Evans, Barer, and Marmor, 1994:50).

Cultural differences, reflected in variation in values and the interpretation of symbols and events, play a key role in the impact of life events on health status (Corin, 1994).

Illness Behavior

"Illness behavior," or responses to what could be the signs and symptoms of a health problem, also plays a role in determining how quickly early health problems are addressed, as well as the effect of such interventions. There are well-known variations between men and women, between young and old people, across ethnic groups, and across socioeconomic status groups in such illness behavior (Cockerham, 1992:97-120; Weiss and Lonnquist, 1994:143-144, 221-244).

A major problem in medical practice is lack of patient compliance with the recommended medical care plan. Noncompliance probably reflects differences in values, beliefs, and cognitive interpretations of the meaning and implications of symptoms, all of which are related to human diversity variables. As Corin noted, "illness experience is not a simple mirror of the disease process. Rather it reflects personal and collective expectations and values; and social and psychological components of that experience can be more powerful determinants of help-seeking behavior, and of actual disability, than biological abnormalities" (1994:113).

Primary Prevention and Health Promotion

In public health, *primary prevention* refers to efforts to prevent the occurrence of health problems as well as very early identification and intervention. This is in contrast to *secondary prevention* aimed at the control and treatment of existing health problems and to *tertiary prevention*, or prevention of secondary disabilities associated with chronic and/or terminal health problems.

Martin Bloom (1987:305-306) spoke of several emerging themes of primary prevention: (1) a systems orientation because of the recognition of multiple interacting "causes" of most health problems; (2) a proactive approach rather than a reactive one; (3) recognition of the need to teach people coping skills, reduce environmental stress, and increase environmental supports; (4) an awareness that, for example, both contraceptives and abortion are "preventive" measures, although introduced at different points in a process; (5) a sense that it is preferable, ethically, to involve individuals in promoting their own health and preventing health problems than to instigate mass actions that affect everyone, with or without their consent.

The recognition of the role of a mixture of biological, psychological, and sociocultural factors in determining health is reflected in the five main "technologies" of primary prevention:

1. Education
2. Social change in the community or society
3. Promotion of competency
4. Promotion of natural caregiving
5. Consultation and collaboration (Gullotta, 1987)

According to Bloom, there is a need to design effective primary prevention strategies that are coordinated and integrated:

Not only must problematic factors be prevented, but promotive factors must be substituted in the system of events in their place. Furthermore, gains at one system level must not be undertaken at the expense of negative changes or losses at other system levels. (1995:1896)

Client Empowerment Orientation

The major causes of death and disability in America today are chronic diseases, for example, heart disease, high blood pressure, cancer, chronic obstructive pulmonary disease (COPD), and diabetes. This is due, in large part, to adverse health behavior, such as smoking; excessive alcohol consumption; too much cholesterol, fat, salt, and sugar in the diet; too few fresh vegetables, fruits, whole grain breads, and cereals, or "roughage"; a lack of physical exercise; and too much "stress."

Client empowerment is key to health promotion and prevention, both to engage individuals in developing healthier lifestyles as well as in becoming active members of the "body politic"—confident and capable of impacting the development of policies and programs of the society to ensure that all its citizens enjoy the social supports they require to realize their full potential.

Although "social support" plays one of the most important roles in mediating/moderating the impact of stressful life events on negative health outcomes, what is perceived as social support varies across and within human diversity variables. For example, persons with a homosexual orientation who are rejected by family and community of origin may develop a "gay community" that functions as a surrogate family. African Americans, whose sense of well-being is often under attack from the external world, employ their church and extended family, including fictive family members, to effectively counteract any harmful impact. This is believed by many to explain why African Americans have a suicide rate half that of white Americans. However, not all African Americans find church to be a source of social support, and not all gays or lesbians are rejected by their families or find support in a "gay community."

In addition, it may be that cultural variables, such as the extent to which a society values individual competition relative to the well-being of the family, group, or community, may be a kind of social support. The extent to which a society provides for its people through "social security" programs, such as are reported to be particularly strong in Scandinavian nations, may also serve as social support.

In short, whatever forces in the social environment cause us to feel cared about and taken care of when needed may be viewed as forms of social support. Social support is empowering. It is an adjunct to our own resources and makes us feel stronger. It may derive from satisfaction with our roles in society, family, work, church, and other community organizations. Wherever it comes from, it makes us feel worthwhile, valued, respected, and secure.

Effective health prevention programs must identify and draw upon cultural and community *strengths* of the client rather than deficits or weaknesses (Green, 1995:227).

INTERDISCIPLINARY TEAMWORK

The need for collaboration across disciplines obviously derives from the theoretical perspective of primary health care. However, as often happens, practice does not always keep pace with theory:

> Some models of primary care include a team of physicians only, some also include representatives of other disciplines, such as nursing, social work, physician extenders, nurse practitioners, and nutritionists. (Miller, 1987:321)

However, Miller also noted:

> to accomplish the goals of the primary care model, the interdisciplinary team is not only desirable but essential. . . . However committed to the biopsychosocial approach, the physician alone cannot be the sole provider. (1987:324)

The Institute of Medicine Committee acknowledges that knowledge of the family and community may also help the primary care clinician better understand the health problems and health risks faced by the patient. In addition, personnel in primary care teams and settings often may be able to act on behalf of their patients in settings and circumstances outside the traditional health environment (Donaldson et al., 1996:59).

ORGANIZATIONAL CONSIDERATIONS

The role and function of social work in primary health care, including public health and primary prevention, will greatly depend on (1) funding sources, (2) whether the host setting of primary care is public tax supported, voluntary nonprofit, or private for profit, (3) and, if private, what, if any, sectarian influence there is.

In addition, the geographical location of the organization in terms of whether rural or urban and the cultural influences in the surrounding community will impact on the social worker role and function.

Funding sources for social work in primary health care settings, depending on the host organization, include Medicare and Medicaid, private health insurance, private out-of-pocket fees, and administrative overhead approaches (Ell and Morrison, 1981:39s).

Another significant organizational variable is by which standard-setting organization it is accredited, if any. The requirements concerning social work services tend to vary and to impact greatly on whether the organization employs social workers, how many it employs, the extent to which social work services are viewed as essential and integrated with the whole program, and the degree requirements for social work services.

CLIENT PROBLEMS
AND SOCIAL WORKER FUNCTIONS

Client Problems

Most of the health problems we face today are substantially caused by destructive human behavior or by ignorance, unrelieved environmental stress, social injustice, and other social or emotional conditions, which are the arena of social workers more than physicians.

Examples of common biopsychosocial health problems requiring social worker participation in treatment include drug and alcohol abuse, child abuse and neglect, domestic violence, elder abuse, teenage pregnancy, sexually transmitted diseases, suicide, depression, homicide, motor vehicle accidents, tobacco addiction, eating disorders such as anorexia, bulimia, and obesity, obsessive-compulsive behaviors, panic disorders, agoraphobia, social isolation, emotional withdrawal, and self-mutilation behavior.

Patients who are obese are at high risk for heart disease, cancer, high blood pressure, and other serious health problems. Yet obesity is probably most often the result of overeating—especially of high-fat, high-cholesterol, high-sugar, and high-salt "comfort foods," compulsively consumed in an effort to relieve long-term underlying emotional pain.

People with mental health problems tend to seek attention for somatic complaints from primary care physicians more than from mental health specialists (Shannon, 1989:35). In much of America, especially among rural people, elderly people, Asian Americans, those of lower socioeconomic status, and certain religious groups, such as Mormons, it is often socially unacceptable to seek help for psychological distress from a mental health professional. As a result, primary care physicians may be used instead, with patients presenting vague or confusing complaints of unclear meaning.

However, most primary care physicians are not trained or motivated to provide direct counseling or psychotherapeutic services and instead tend to rely on pharmaceutical interventions, which often bring short-term symptom relief without problem relief. Cassell, a famous physician, presents his vision for future medical education that will produce doctors who can competently and confidently address the psychosocial problems of primary care patients, claiming such changes in medical education are necessary because "It is not uncommon to find graduating medical students who have had no training in normal or abnormal psychology, no experience with nondrug treatment of emotional illness, and no instruction in the psychology of physical illness" (1995:385).

Social Worker Functions

The functions of social work in a public health program include the following:

1. Participating in the planning and implementation of programs for the protection of communities from health hazards, the promotion of improved personal health care, and the prevention of ill health, including the promotion of positive health behaviors

2. Use of the epidemiologic approach in determining the association between social factors and the incidence of health problems and planning intervention strategies to promote health, protect against specific diseases, provide early intervention, prevent avoidable disability, and maximize comfort and function of impaired persons
3. Alleviation of social stress associated with having health problems and utilization of social supports to promote well-being and health protection
4. Participation in outreach to at-risk persons to ensure access to health care and needed social services
5. Participation in promoting consumer involvement and leadership in the planning and delivery of health care and relevant social services. (NASW, 1987:12-14)

Thus, it would appear from the NASW standards that, depending on the population using primary care services, social workers may be engaged in program planning and policy formulation, community needs assessment, outreach to members of high-risk populations, health education to individuals and groups, formation and facilitation of self-help groups, and conducting epidemiological research to identify high-risk groups (Miller, 1987:322).

However, most social workers in primary health care are in direct service roles, providing clients with counseling and linkage to community resources (Green and Kulper, 1990; Oktay, 1984). For example, social workers in primary care may provide appropriate services to address the psychosocial needs of patients who would otherwise present somatic complaints and misuse primary medical care. In the medical clinic of an urban hospital adjacent to an impoverished African-American community, a group of social workers reported on their interesting project to empower patients through the social support of the group (Dobrof et al., 1990). According to the authors, the groups were effective, both in reducing physical symptomatology and in engaging clients in a more active role in their own health care. The social workers saw themselves as role models, facilitators, teachers, skill builders, and change promoters (Dobrof et al., 1990:36).

Eight groups were developed to address specific psychosocial problems:

1. A men's stress management group for those with anxiety leading to psychosomatic symptoms
2. An empty nest syndrome group for middle-aged women who need to discover life outside the empty nest
3. Senior socialization for isolated elder women
4. Support groups for people with a common physical disease
5. Support groups for people with a common psychiatric disorder
6. A housing advocacy group to teach people how to self-advocate to get action on environmental issues (Dobrof et al., 1990)

Most social workers continue to seem to prefer clinical social work with individuals and to lack interest in, and/or knowledge of, more macro-level interventions. In one study of social workers in the primary care setting of family practice residency programs (Hess, 1985), the social workers reported that most of the patients had a cluster of psychosocial problems rather than just one, and the problems identified covered a wide range of types. However, the social workers were selective in their choice of which client problems to address:

> Respondent's descriptions of their clinical work conveyed a general tendency to select emotional/interpersonal conflict client problems rather than social/environmental problems; interventions within the therapeutic type; and an individual rather than a family, agency, or community focus. (Hess, 1985:60)

In addition, in the Hess study (1985), many of the social workers were engaged in educating the physicians through their clinical practice. However, since the social workers tended to self-select a limited type of client problem rather than making a representative selection of the clients' actual problems, the implication is that their teaching of the physicians would also tend to present a biased picture, one preoccupied with emotional and individual problems, to the exclusion of social environmental and family-centered ones (Hess, 1985:61-62).

Zayas and Dyche (1992) describe their social work practice in a primary care medical clinic and residency program, where they teach physicians about attending to four main, essentially clinical concepts:

1. The concept of process (development of events), including beginning "where the patient is" in their concerns and interpretations
2. The helping relationship and "conscious use of self"
3. The person-in-situation perspective (what is going on in the patient's life situation when the health complaints ebb and flow)
4. The context of practice (from the clinical setting to the community, home, school, workplace, as well as the patient's own demographic characteristics)

Constraints on Social Work in Primary Health Care

According to Miller (1987:323), barriers to social worker participation in primary health care include the following: (1) physicians lack understanding of the knowledge, functions, and skills of social workers and of the biopsychosocial model; (2) as primary care becomes competitive, a challenge may emerge for primary care practitioners in medicine to retain a large enough patient load, thus providing a disincentive to employ people such as social workers who could effectively contribute to health promotion and the prevention of health problems; (3) most primary care will probably be provided through HMOs, which are likely to serve a predominately economically comfortable sector of the population, which the medical staff may not perceive as needing social work services. Yet another barrier to social worker involvement in primary health care may be social workers' lack of educational preparation for this type of work (Oktay, 1995:1891).

Furthermore, there has been a general lack of funding for social work in primary care. Most health insurance plans provide minimal coverage for mental health services or for preventive services in general. With the current focus on cost control, case management service (assessment, referral, and coordination of services to be provided by others) is more likely to be funded than direct provision of needed services (Oktay, 1995:1892).

A still greater barrier to social work in primary care may be the lack of qualified social workers, especially in rural areas. In 1985, the Task Force on Social Services in Primary Care was organized to study a sample of both rural and urban community health centers funded through Section 330 of the U.S. Public Health Service Act and ascertain the use of, and need for, social work services in these centers (Young and Martin, 1989). They found that although the patients were reported to have many of the same types of social problems in both rural and urban centers, the social work support available to address them was different. The rural centers employed far fewer social workers for the size of the patient load and also hired far fewer MSW-level social workers, even to direct the social work program, and rural centers made fewer referrals to community resources other than hospitals. Many of the rural primary care centers were staffed by only one BSW-level social worker to handle all the psychosocial problems presented.

However, primary care practice of physicians varies between rural and urban areas in its use of social worker assistance. While rural primary care physicians are unlikely to employ social workers to assist with addressing patients' psychosocial problems, social work practice in primary care is much more common in urban areas. Some study of rural primary care physicians to explore their current and potential use of social workers indicates that they tend to perceive social workers as specializing in resource referral and linkage tasks (Badger et al., 1997). This was also the finding of an earlier study of physicians' and nurses' perceptions of the hospital social worker role (Cowles and Lefcowitz, 1995).

There is unquestioned need for qualified social workers in primary health care. A recent study of the extent to which primary care physicians encounter psychosocial problems of patients found that primary care physicians are, indeed, the "gatekeepers" for an array of psychosocial problems (Gross et al., 1996:89). Zayas and Dyche (1992) expect increased federal funding for primary care, including increased demand for social workers, whose functions would include a greater role in medical education.

KNOWLEDGE REQUIREMENTS

Given the complex theoretical perspective of primary care in the health field and the associated necessity of interdisciplinary teamwork, various areas of knowledge are required for optimal social work practice in primary care.

Ell and Morrison wrote, "the social worker in a primary health care setting is truly a generalist and must be prepared to intervene at many levels—individual, family, group, or community" (1981:37s). They continue:

> the knowledge base in primary care social work is unique in its breadth. The array of medical and emotional problems presented in different primary care settings requires social workers to have an unusually extensive knowledge of medicine, psychopathology, and organizational theory. Knowledge of epidemiology, the etiology of illness, psychosocial dysfunction, and the sociology of medicine provides the foundation for decisions about which patients to treat and with what technology. (Ell and Morrison, 1981:37s)

A Model Curriculum for Social Work in Primary Care

A model primary care curriculum for schools of social work and other professional schools to adopt is recommended by the Michigan Prevention Training and Curriculum Development Project, explaining that

> The Public Health Social Work Forward Plan documents the need for graduate schools of social work to incorporate increased public health content into their curricula to prepare practitioners to work in a broad range of practice settings beyond those traditionally associated with public health. (Siefert, Jayaratne, and Martin, 1992:18)

The following principles provide the foundation for the recommended curriculum:

1. health and mental health conceptualized holistically as positive well-being, not merely the absence of disease;
2. a developmental perspective emphasizing competence and mastery as well as vulnerability over the life cycle;
3. knowledge of the impact of individual and environmental risk factors in the etiology and prevention of health and mental health disorders;

4. an understanding of the protective function of social support;
5. concepts and strategies from epidemiology;
6. comprehension of research design and methodology appropriate to prevention; and
7. appreciation of the need to intervene at multiple levels using a range of preventive strategies. (Siefert, Jayaratne, and Martin, 1992:19)

The proposed curriculum plan has been integrated with the Council on Social Work Education's required core curriculum of human behavior and the social environment, social welfare policy and services, social work practice, social work research methods, and field practicum (Siefert, Jayaratne, and Martin, 1992:19). One of the most interesting aspects of the proposed curriculum is that the participating graduate students are required to design a social work intervention project aimed at prevention and to test its effect (Siefert, Jayaratne, and Martin, 1992:22).

Need for Conceptual Integration
of Physical and Mental Health

In addition, the proposal challenges schools of social work to recognize that the traditional separation of health and mental health is no longer workable (Siefert, Jayaratne, and Martin, 1992:25). Shannon also wrote:

> A biopsychosocial model of health care—in which disease is seen as an interplay between environmental, physical, behavioral, psychological, and social factors—can integrate mental health services into the primary care sector (1989:32).

Tessie Cleveland added:

> The historical division between medical social work and psychiatric social work has been serious and divisive, perpetuating a caste system within the social work profession. . . . Social workers have not yet recognized forthrightly that the division, which may serve some ego needs, confuses colleagues outside social work and undermines the profession. . . . Social workers

must move to present uniform definitions of health and mental health practice and must seek reform in social work education and agency administration to solidify this uniformity. Social workers should be proud that . . . they can maintain a single identity and view the client holistically. To this end, each disease . . . with its accompanying psychosocial involvement, has import for social work practice. (1981:125)

The Need to Move Beyond Clinical Social Work

Addressing the subject of "prevention," Pray (1995) noted that the trend today in national and international places with progressive health care approaches is to focus on community organization and community empowerment and policy changes, which go beyond one-on-one efforts to modify health behavior. Pray cites Bracht (1990) as a rich source of information about such projects.

This suggests that schools of social work must make a greater effort to lure future social workers from a preoccupation with one-on-one clinical work to greater interest and competency in community organization and social action approaches.

Need for Collaboration Between Classroom and Practicum

Finally, to develop the necessary knowledge and skills for effective social work practice in health care, it is imperative that social work education in the classroom and field practicum employs coordinated and cooperative educational efforts. These efforts should include (1) the classroom and practicum exchanging information concerning their curriculum content and changes; (2) classroom faculty providing field faculty with written descriptions of areas of concentration, course descriptions, and research programs; (3) field instructors providing classroom faculty with information about their agency programs, field curricula, and seminar presentations; (4) more joint programs between the two to exchange information and and share ideas; and (5) seminars by the schools for field instructors to promote information exchange between agencies and between agencies and schools (Marshack, Davidson, and Mizrahi, 1988:231).

Summary

Ideally then, social work practice in primary care in the health field requires knowledge of the following: health behavior, illness behavior, social aspects of illness, generalist practice (including how to work at all social systems levels of person, family, group, organization, community, and society), medicine, psychopathology, organizational theory, epidemiology, the etiology of illness, psychosocial dysfunction, the sociology of medicine, the World Health Organization's concept of health, empowerment and the strengths perspective, individual and environmental risk factors, the protective function of social support, epidemiology, experimental research methodology to test the effect of interventions, and the biopsychosocial model of health care.

As stated in Chapter 2, the health care social worker requires specific knowledge in the areas of client population and problem, organizational setting, the community and its resources, specific intervention modalities, and specific methods of research, evaluation, and documentation appropriate to the setting.

VALUES AND ETHICS CONSIDERATIONS

More than any other area of health care, primary care, in the sense of primary prevention and health promotion, must attend to adverse social environmental conditions. According to the current NASW Code of Ethics:

> The *primary mission* of the social work profession is to enhance human well-being and help meet the basic human needs of all people with particular attention to the needs and empowerment of people who are vulnerable, oppressed, and living in poverty. . . . Fundamental to social work is *attention to environmental forces* that create, contribute to, and address problems in living. Social workers promote *social justice and social change* with and on behalf of clients. "Clients" is used inclusively to refer to individuals, families, groups, organizations, and communities. (emphasis added) (NASW, 1996:1)

Social justice is listed as one of the six core values of the social work profession, whose associated ethical principle is stated as follows:

> Social workers *challenge social injustice*. Social workers *pursue social change*, particularly with and on behalf of vulnerable and oppressed individuals and groups of people. Social workers' social change efforts are focused primarily on issues of poverty, unemployment, discrimination, and other forms of social injustice. These activities seek *to promote sensitivity to and knowledge about oppression and cultural ethnic diversity*. Social workers strive *to ensure access to needed information, services, and resources, equality of opportunity, and meaningful participation in decision making for all people*. (emphasis added) (NASW, 1996:5)

Given the organizational pressures that increasingly are felt by all professionals in health care settings today to compromise their values and ethics, it is important for social workers to remember that their responsibilities begin with *a primary responsibility to promote their clients' well-being* "In general, *the clients' interests are primary*" (emphasis added) (NASW, 1996:7).

In addition, the social worker has an *obligation to promote the client's right to self-determination and to understand and respect the client's culture and social diversity* (NASW, 1996:7, 9).

SKILL REQUIREMENTS

Ell and Morrison (1981) listed among the skills needed by social workers in primary health care decision making, differential diagnosis, counseling the resistant patient, team building, consultation, and education. Other needed social work skill areas include case finding, discriminating between various biopsychosocial sources of patient anxiety, the ability to help some patients recognize the source of their symptoms as social or emotional rather than organic, facilitating the learning and application of psychosocial assessment and treatment skills by other professions in addition to social work, and teaching skills, especially about how to interview and about how psychosocial issues affect health and illness. Primary care social workers also need to be skilled in the use of community resources for health promotion and prevention of health problems, such as referring primary care clients to particular programs, for example, weight control, cessation of smoking, Alcoholics Anonymous, support groups, and training in such skills as effective parenting, self-assertion, nutrition, and child development.

Research and evaluation skills are also needed by social workers, especially in primary care, to develop tools for assessing clients' need for social work services so that referrals to social work are not limited to the physician's judgment of need (Ell and Morrison, 1981:38s).

Finally, research skills are needed to evaluate practice in order to refine primary care social work practice by developing knowledge concerning what are and are not effective social work interventions in primary health care. By so doing, social workers can develop credibility and gain funding to support the work.

Hess examined social work practice in a primary care setting and concluded that

> . . . social work graduate education needs to strengthen its ability to promote excellence in areas of teaching, health care coordination, and health team participation, [as well as in] areas of physical illness, health behavior, and social aspects of illness, [in addition to] methodology for work with families. [Note that] *an effective practice model of social work in primary health care settings is needed.* (emphasis added) (1985:64)

HELPING INTERVENTIONS

Ell and Morrison noted the following about social work interventions in primary health care settings:

> Interventions used with patients include evaluation, information and referral, outreach, case management, short-term psychotherapy, family and group therapy, crisis intervention, family planning, genetic counseling, behavior modification, patient edu-

cation, and facilitating and advocating system or community development and change. Interventions with [interdisciplinary] teams include consultation, staff development, in-service education, administrative analysis, and professional research. (1981:37s)

Bloom (1995) suggests a variety of potential interventions for social workers to use in primary prevention work at the micro level, such as problem-solving, coping, and social skills, self-efficacy development, assertiveness training, cognitive reframing, anticipatory coping, parent effectiveness training, and social support groups.

Although such interventions would doubtlessly help, they do not address the adverse social institutional conditions that seem to be at the root of poor health, such as social inequality and unequal opportunity, illuminated by Evans, Barer, and Marmor (1994) and Kozol (1991, 1995).

The Need for Macro-Level Change

Social workers will not be able to change the economic system, educational system, political system, or health care system unless they become more involved in community organization and other macro-level approaches directed to empowering the public (Dunlop and Holosko, 1992).

The public must be engaged in demanding a dramatic reduction in both absolute and relative poverty, the development of national health insurance or some other national health care system that ensures access to primary medical care, and more early identification of, and intervention in, family and community situations that threaten the mental and physical well-being of their members. Only then will it be possible to prevent the damage to human development that results in behavior that is destructive to self and others:

The philosophy of primary health care emphasizes prevention, health education, community participation (not token, but listening to all local viewpoints with respect), the importance of environmental factors, and the need to reach out to even the most remote areas and to all parts of the population, including the poorest. (Smyre, 1993:59)

Social Mapping

All intervention in primary care must be rooted in sensitivity to human diversity. Community participation, community organization work, must employ what Cochane (1979, cited in Green, 1995:100) termed "social mapping," a kind of inventory at the macro-social level, including:

1. Identification and location of an ethnic group in an area
2. Description of the community's social organization
3. Description of the residents' beliefs and ideological character- istics
4. Identification of patterns of wealth, its accumulation, and its distribution
5. Description of the patterns of mobility, both geographical and social
6. Information on access and utilization of available human ser- vices

Green wrote the following about the result of social mapping:

The product of social mapping should be a short document containing one or more physical maps and descriptive infor- mation for each of the six items listed above, provided in sufficient detail that a stranger could read it and gain some general sense of: (a) who lives in the area; (b) how they live; (c) what they believe and do; (d) how they use social services. The document should also make clear the outstanding needs of the community, especially as they are perceived by the resi- dents themselves. (1995:100-101)

Caring at the Primary Health Care Level

Caring at the primary health care level is directed at primary prevention and health promotion. It is comparable to the nurture of children or plants or anything else we value and wish to do well. It means that we must determine what is needed in order to do well, and then we must assume responsibility for providing the proper care. In other words, "caring" is rooted in *caring about* something, but is relatively meaningless unless we assume responsibility to ensure that needs are met. To do otherwise is "careless."

Therefore, it seems careless for a society to ignore the social conditions that are adverse to the prevention of health problems and the promotion of health. It is this writer's conviction that the entire field of social work in health care needs to awaken to the social structural conditions in the etiology of health problems. For example:

- A society is not "healthy" if 20 percent of its children are without economic means to live according to even minimal standards of decency and health.
- A society is not "healthy" if it relies on the local property tax base as the primary source of public school funding, which results in vast differences in the quality of public education from one locality to another.
- A society is not "healthy" if the percentage of its citizens incarcerated in prisons and jails is the highest in the world.
- A society is not "healthy" if 15 percent of its members have no health insurance, despite the majority of them being employed full-time.
- A society is not "healthy" if over 50 percent of its citizens who are poor, according to its own poverty index, are not covered by its Medicaid health insurance program for the poor.
- A society is not "healthy" if its own low standard for distinguishing the poor from the nonpoor is itself considerably higher than the legally required minimum wage.
- A society is not "healthy" if its government will not allocate enough funds to employ a sufficient number of adequately trained staff to competently address the problems of physical, emotional, and sexual child maltreatment.
- A society is not "healthy" if it so morally insensitive that it allows its federal Congress members to have comprehensive health insurance, while these same persons fail to enact policy providing the same to the rest of the citizenry.

- A society is not "healthy" if it claims to be the "best in the world" and yet continues to be the only industrialized nation in the world without any system of national health care, and still claims that medical care ought to be purchased from providers who are in the business primarily to make a profit.
- A society is not "healthy" if it attempts to achieve cost control in health care through a system that allows the chief executive officers of managed health care organizations to receive multimillion-dollar annual incomes from the profits derived from withholding needed medical interventions to their patients.
- A society is not "healthy" if its Congress does not take legislative action to ensure that Medicare reimbursement to medical supply companies is based on competitive bids, as is done in the Veterans Administration, but instead continues to allow the Health Care Financing Administration to pay claims, without challenge, which are sometimes hundreds of times higher than over-the-counter costs, because the Congress has succumbed to the lobbying and political contributions of this supply industry, and seeks, instead, to compensate for this total waste of taxpayer money by increasing out-of-pocket cost sharing of elderly and disabled Medicare recipients.

The major danger for the future of primary health care in the United States is that the goal of cost control will be achieved through using public funds and legislative policy to promote a profit-making industry that will be extremely lucrative to stockholders and CEOs. This will cause the general public in America to experience a reduction in the quality and quantity of health services and make members of the medical profession salaried employees of business and industry. As a result, the health of the nation will continue to decline.

Perhaps social work in health care in the twenty-first century needs to consider a return to settlement house social work as practiced at the turn of the twentieth century, as described at the beginning of this chapter.

CONCLUSION

Hopefully, the U.S. health care system will finally realize that the only effective route to cost control is through greater focus on primary prevention of health problems—thoroughly rooted in addressing the underlying social problems of poverty, racism, environmental pollution, lack of education, and general lack of "caring" for ourselves and one another.

This recognition will mark the end of what has often been referred to as "the medicalization of social problems." When this awakening happens, social workers will be employed as one of the important groups of agents needed to achieve the goals of primary care.

Chapter 4

Social Work in Hospitals

HISTORICAL BACKGROUND

The Development of Hospitals in the United States

Originally, hospitals in the United States were almshouses for the poor, and many of them later became well-known, public tax-supported hospitals. For example, Bellevue Hospital in New York City was founded in 1736 as the second almshouse in the country. The first almshouse was established in Philadelphia in 1713 (Nacman, 1977:407).

During the second half of the 1700s, private nonprofit hospitals began to emerge, on demand of the middle class, who saw the need for hospitals but were repelled by the squalor of the almshouses. One reason for their emergence at this time was the need for treatment facilities for those injured in the Revolutionary War (Nacman, 1977:408).

After the Revolutionary War, immigration and urbanization increased and were accompanied by epidemics and other public health problems (Rosen, 1958:182, 201). Consequently, more public hospitals were built, such as Massachusetts General in 1821 and the Lincoln Hospital in 1840, built in New York City for the care of elderly and disabled African Americans (Nacman, 1977:408).

However, even by the mid-1800s, almshouses continued as centers of care for most of the economically and otherwise dependent population. Recognition was spreading, though, that the conditions in almshouses were extremely bad, and specialized care facilities began to emerge for subgroups seen as "deserving" of being saved from almshouses—such as children, the elderly, and the mentally ill and developmentally disabled. Thus, society saw the growth of orphanages, homes for the aged (often for specific religious or ethnic groups), and state hospitals for the mentally ill and developmentally disabled (Nacman, 1977). In addition, there arose "outdoor" relief assistance programs, in cash or in kind, also to save specific religious or ethnic group members from almshouses.

Although the first hospitals emerged in the second half of the 1700s, they did not become the center of medical practice until around the end of the 1800s, when the germ theory of disease began to be widely accepted (Cannon, 1923).

The Emergence of Social Work

The need developed for some system to oversee and set standards for these new institutional care facilities, as well as to coordinate the multiple outdoor relief charities that were emerging. The people who filled these positions on the State Boards of Charities and Corrections and with the Charity Organization Societies later came to perceive themselves as having a common function and philosophy, and they adopted the title "social worker." Settlement house staff were the third set of new workers responding to similar conditions.

Social Work in the Health Care Field

Social work in the health care field is usually traced to the entry of social work into the general hospital. However, from the time social work emerged in the mid-1800s, its practitioners were involved with the multiple health-related problems of poverty, overcrowding, and the lack of proper water and sewage systems that accompanied urbanization and immigration, unregulated and unplanned industrialization, and lack of acceptance of the emerging germ theory of disease (Rosen, 1958:348-349, 353, 360-364; Trattner, 1989:133-134).

Growth of Hospital Social Work

In 1984, there were 6,872 hospitals in the United States, of which 6,302 (92 percent) responded to an annual survey of the American

Hospital Association (AHA). Of the 6,302 that responded, 5,209, or 83 percent, reported having social work services. Of the reporting hospitals, 5,801 were general and nonpsychiatric speciality hospitals, and about 82 percent of these had social work services. The remaining 501 reporting hospitals in 1984 were psychiatric hospitals, and 95 percent of them had social work services (American Hospital Association, 1985).

In 1994, there were 6,374 hospitals in the United States, of which 5,387 (84.5 percent) responded to an annual survey of the American Hospital Association. Of those which responded, 4,707, (87 percent) reported having social work services. Of the total reporting hospitals in 1994, 4,926 (77 percent) were general and nonpsychiatric specialty hospitals, and 4,350 (88 percent) of these had social work services. The remaining 461 reporting hospitals in 1994 were psychiatric hospitals, and 357 (77 percent) of them had social work services (American Hospital Association, 1997). Table 4.1 depicts this comparison.

TABLE 4.1. Number and Percentage of Reporting Hospitals with Social Work Services, 1984 and 1994

Reporting Hospitals	Hospitals with Social Work Services			
	1984 Number	1984 Percent	1994 Number	1994 Percent
Psychiatric specialty hospitals N = 501 (1984) N = 461 (1994)	478	95	357	77
General/nonpsychiatric specialty hospitals N = 5801 (1984) N = 4926 (1994)	4731	82	4350	88
Total hospitals N = 6302 (1984) N = 5387 (1994)	5209	83	4707	87

Sources: American Hospital Association (1985). Phone conversation between author and an AHA spokesperson, Chicago, April; American Hospital Association (1997). AHA Resource Center, data derived from AHA *1995 Annual Survey.* Data faxed to author from Mark Barbaree.

The U.S. Department of Labor estimated that, in 1992, a total of 26.2 percent of social workers were employed in the health care field, and 14.13 percent alone were employed in hospitals, both public and private, by far the largest employer of social workers in health care (Ginsberg, 1995:355).

THEORETICAL PERSPECTIVES

Curing

When the germ theory of disease began to be widely accepted, medical practice recognized the desirability of aseptic conditions for surgery and wound care, and the possibility of preventing and "curing" infection through antiseptic was not demonstrated until 1867, when Joseph Lister, a surgeon, did so (Rosen, 1958:317). However, it was not until the last decade of the 19th century and the first decade of the twentieth century that the germ theory of disease was well-developed and accepted (319).

The modern hospital became the seat of medical practice when this was occurring, and it began a transition from *social medicine* to the *medical model*, and from *caring* to *curing*. Indeed, the hope of conquering human disease grew ever larger during the twentieth century, eventually resulting in a hospital-centered health care system whose costs of high technology and specialization were rising so much faster than those of other industries that the U.S. government began to take steps to reduce the use of hospitals and medical specialists.

Cost-Effectiveness

Cost control became the overriding concern of U.S. hospitals as the health care inflation rate rose from 5.1 percent of the GDP (gross domestic product) in 1960, to 7.1 percent in 1970, to 8 percent in 1980, to 12.1 percent in 1990, and to 13.6 percent in 1993. The United States expends both a higher per capita amount and a higher percentage of its GDP on health care than any other country in the world, including those with national health care systems (U.S. Government Printing Office, 1995a:240).

National health expenditures totaled $949.4 billion in 1994 in the United States; the largest percentage of the total, 35.7 percent, or $338.9 billion, went for hospital care (U.S. Government Printing Office, 1995a:244). Only since the DRG system went into effect in 1984 has the annual rate of increase begun to decline. While from 1975 to 1980 it peaked at 14.3 percent, from 1980 to 1985 it dropped to 10.4, and from 1993 to 1994, it declined to an annual rate of only a 4.4 percent increase (U.S. Government Printing Office, 1995a:244).

Of the total expended for hospitalization in 1994, 78.2 percent went to general medical hospitals, 12.1 percent to psychiatric hospitals, and the remaining 9.7 percent to other specialty hospitals (U.S. Government Printing Office, 1995b:table 178, 122). The financing of hospital care in 1994, including hospital-based nursing home and home health agency care, is shown in Table 4.2.

TABLE 4.2. Financing Hospital Care, 1994

Government 59.0%	
30.0 % Medicare	
14.6 % Medicaid	
14.4 % Other government programs, such as VA, and state and local government subsidies to hospitals	
Private health insurance 34.2%	
Out-of-pocket payments 2.9%	
Other private funds 4.0%	
Total ($338.5 billion) 100.1%	

Source: U.S. Government Printing Office (1995a). *Health, United States.* Washington, DC: Author, 250.

The Biopsychosocial Model

Since at least the beginning of hospital social work, social workers have recognized that biological, psychological, and social environmental variables impact one another. The *mission of social work in the acute-care medical hospital* is delineated by the National Association of Social Workers (1990) as follows:

Social work services are provided to patients and their families to meet their medically related social and emotional needs as they impinge on their medical condition, treatment, and recovery, and safe transition from one care environment to another. (NASW, 1990:4)

However, the focus of hospital social work has tended to shift back and forth between "psychological," "social," and "psychosocial" as the profession as a whole responded to changing professional and national political priorities. Thus, hospital social work started in 1905 with a social medicine view of the social roots of health problems when infectious and contagious diseases were predominant. In the 1920s, social work shifted to a Freudian view of individual-seated problems, in search of achievement of Abraham Flexnor's concept of "professional status," to which the medical profession had already succumbed by shifting from a social medicine perspective to the medical model (Smith and Anderson, 1995:248).

During the 1930s, the focus of social work moved to an acknowledgment of the force of macro-level political and economic conditions, as the suicide rate skyrocketed and the general population ate at soup kitchens during the Great Depression.

In the euphoric era of post-World War II, social work again moved back to a more individual-centered approach.

Then, during the social justice and antimaterialistic period of the 1960s and 1970s, hospital social work moved back to a more social action orientation.

Finally during the conservative backlash of the 1980s, social work again returned to a more individual focus, where it and society generally remain lodged. While lip service is given to "psychosocial," the emphasis appears mostly to be on the "psycho" part—less as a result of conviction than from a sense of powerlessness, perhaps.

Unfortunately, this early lack of consensus concerning the focus of hospital social work and the profession in general led to a division within the profession, creating a separation between "medical" and "psychiatric" social workers, so that throughout much of this century of hospital social work, many hospitals maintained separate social work departments, one a department of medical social work and the other a department of psychiatric social work, despite their role and function being more alike than different (Nacman, 1977).

Caring

Caring at the "acute," that is, secondary level of health care, refers to providing needed assistance to support comfort and function while the person is temporarily impaired by illness or injury to enhance or facilitate the curative or recovery process. Such care interventions may be directed to either physical, psychological, or social comfort and function aspects by addressing (1) barriers to admission to the hospital; (2) problems of adjustment to the hospital; (3) problems adjusting to the diagnosis, prognosis, or treatment plan; (4) lack of information to make informed decisions and to feel in control; (5) lack of resources to meet needs; and (6) barriers to discharge.

HUMAN DIVERSITY RELEVANCE

As indicated elsewhere, human diversity variables, such as age, gender, ethnicity, sexual orientation, disability, rural or urban residence, religion, and social class, can influence health behavior, illness behavior, and sick-role behavior and can interact rather than being merely additive. That is, one cannot assume that within each group people are alike, and so the traits of a "typical female" can merely be combined with those of a "typical elderly person" and a "typical African-American person," for example. Instead, females differ across class, ethnicity, sexual orientation, age, health status, and so on. Likewise, African Americans differ across class, gender, age, health status, and sexual orientation, and so forth. Nonetheless, the hospital social worker needs to have some familiarity with broad health-related differences across class (income, education, and occupation), ethnicity, gender, age group, and so on, yet not assume that such differences are true of all members of a particular group.

A recent and excellent text dealing with ethnicity and health care is *Multicultural Awareness in the Health Care Professions* (Julia, 1996).

It is always important for the hospital social worker to understand the client's view of the nature of his or her health problem, its causes and effects, and the appropriate treatment. Otherwise, the client may simply appear to agree, when, in reality, he or she has another perspective and plan. Of course, this difference in perspective may be due to a discrepancy in any one or a combination of variables, such as values, beliefs, customs, attitudes, resources, experience, or simply understanding.

African-American Health Beliefs

Congress and Lyons have discussed some of the cultural differences in health beliefs and their implications for social work in health care settings. They point out that part of the African-American tradition includes the conceptualization of health problems as falling into three categories: natural, occult, and spiritual (1992:83), with associated intervention types. For example, natural illness was often treated with herbal remedies, occult health disorders with witchcraft or "rootwork," and spiritual problems with prayer and the laying on of hands (Ibid.). Black Americans of Haitian origin may attribute their health problems to supernatural causes and employ voodoo interventions.

Hispanic-American Health Beliefs

On the other hand, Hispanic-American people tend to think of health problems as either "natural" ones that God has willed or "unnatural" ones that other people have caused through evil intent (Congress and Lyons, 1992:84). In either case, the idea that individuals have the power to greatly influence their own health through health behaviors may be outside the belief system of Hispanic-American persons. Hispanic-Americans see mind and body as a unity and "health" as dependent upon harmony with one's social and physical environment; thus, their emotional problems tended to manifest as somatic complaints (85).

The description of symptoms and interpretation of the health problem that the Hispanic-American patient or family member gives the health care provider may be misleading, if the provider is unaware of these kinds of cultural differences. Hispanic-American people of Puerto Rican background may seek assistance from a folk healer or spiritualist before a physician, and it may be more beneficial to the patient for both traditions to be included in treatment (Congress and Lyons, 1992:85).

Asian-American Health Care Beliefs

There is much diversity within the Asian-American population due to the many different countries and cultures of origin, although many utilize home remedies and believe in a yin-yang food group system (Congress and Lyons, 1992:86).

Similar to Hispanic people, the Chinese tend to express their mental health problems somatically and to describe them in physical terms (Congress and Lyons, 1992:86). However, as with all ethnic groups, their traditions are more often found among the older generation and among those who are less assimilated into U.S. mainstream culture. In addition, people of lower socioeconomic status are more likely to seek informal family and folk remedies, partly because they are more accessible financially. As the Clemens (1995) study of hospital social worker discharge planning with an elderly ethnic population found, "the poor, and especially the ethnic poor, are particularly vulnerable to paternalistic interventions" (Congress and Lyons, 1992:89).

Whenever any patient has preferences for care which are important to them but which deviate from the hospital's usual approach, effort should be made to accommodate them, as long as it does not pose a significant threat to the functioning of the hospital or the well-being of the patient. Examples include food, clothing, or bathing preferences, religious ceremonies, or having loved ones nearby. Presumably, such accommodations can affect the patient's mental attitude, will to live, and sense of social support and empowerment.

INTERDISCIPLINARY TEAMWORK

Ross (1993) has argued that "Our claim to a place on the interdisciplinary team must be based on expertise. Communication with other providers about issues related to patient and family adjustment requires more than a shallow grasp of biopsychosocial aspects of an illness (1993:245).

A key to survival in hospital social work is learning to collaborate and cooperate with other professional groups in the setting in such a way that you complement rather than compete with one another (Ruster, 1995).

However, the problem of a lack of clear role identity within the hospital social worker community has become compounded in recent years by indications that hospital physicians and nurses also have increasingly moved away from the medical model and toward a biopsychosocial perspective (Cowles and Lefcowitz, 1992). This appears to have led to increased overlapping of roles among professional groups in interdisciplinary teamwork. For example, Cowles and Lefcowitz, in their study of interdisciplinary expectations of the hospital social worker role, found that at least 60 percent of the physicians and nurses expected to at least equally share with other professional groups, such as social workers, responsibility for the assessment of both emotional and social environmental problems of their patients and for helping patients examine solutions to their emotional problems (1992:63).

As Donnelly (1992) pointed out:

> Under the impact of the knowledge explosion, increasing members of the interdisciplinary team share a common knowledge base (108). . . . Nurses, psychologists, physicians as well as a growing variety of counselors and therapists have often read the same books, undergone similar training and share many of the same skills as social workers . . . [in short] the psychosocial [arena] is by no means the exclusive domain of social workers (109).

Still, recent research has also found considerable interdisciplinary concensus concerning the expected roles and functions of physicians, nurses, and social workers in urban hospitals (Cowles and Lefcowitz, 1992, 1995) and between nurses and social workers in rural hospitals (Egan and Kadushin, 1995). The main difference is a tendency for social workers to expect more *exclusive* responsibility for assessing patients' emotional problems, while the other professional groups expect this to be a task that is shared.

There is growing recognition today that responsibility for addressing psychosocial needs of patients and families is not confined to any one professional group. This is reflected in an excellent article by Lauria and colleagues, who published a protocol for "clinicians charged with providing psychosocial care" (1996:1345) to child cancer patients and their families. The article offers a conceptualization of a systematic process of examining and helping with common psychosocial needs of child cancer patients and their families at various stages of disease course, for use by a multidisciplinary team of specialists in cancer care, including a pediatric oncologist, oncology nurses, oncology social workers, and pediatric psychologists (1347). The article provides an outline for the psychosocial assessment of both patient and family as well as an extensive list (protocol) of client issues and needs and associated clinical interventions that are relevant at various stages in the course of the child cancer condition.

ORGANIZATIONAL CONSIDERATIONS

Politically Conservative Hospital Roots

Hospitals tend to be conservative organizations, especially today, when more are for profit, but the medical profession has always been dominant in hospitals and its members have traditionally derived from an upper-middle-class conservative perspective. Medical practice addresses health problems in individuals, not adverse social conditions that may have produced the health problems.

The Challenge to Hospital Social Workers

Thus, the organizational environment of the hospital tends to produce a culture of conservativism, which is difficult to ignore and survive. Social workers in hospitals need to recognize this influence in order to try to resist it when appropriate. Otherwise, the social worker is likely to become a "tool" of the system—resulting in becoming an agent for facilitating hospital and medical professional survival goals and objectives, at the expense of both client (patient and family) health and well-being and social work professional values, ethics, and autonomy—without which, professional status is questionable.

Social work students preparing for hospital social work need to be taught how to set limits in carrying out institutional policies in order to avoid compromising professional autonomy and responsibility (Kadushin and Kulys, 1995:184).

Intraorganizational Variation in Culture

However, hospitals vary, not only from one another, but across intraorganizational units. Each medical and surgical service tends to have a "culture" of its own, reflecting a mixture of variation in characteristics of the health conditions served, the interventions provided, the usual prognosis, and patient and staff characteristics. For example, pediatric and obstetric units are likely to differ considerably in culture from cardiac care and oncology units (James and Studs, 1987).

Vertical Integration of the Modern Hospital

Robinson (1994) said:

> The delivery system of the 21st century might remain centered around the hospital, albeit a vertically integrated system where acute care beds play only a modest role (259). . . . Hospitals have integrated rapidly into outpatient facilities that diagnose patients prior to admission, into subacute care facilities that shelter patients after discharge, and into many forms of health care that are not directly linked to acute inpatient care at all. (262)

Increasingly, community hospital social work departments are achieving recognition by expanding into areas where they are needed and can complement rather than compete with other professions and health care organizations. These areas include joint nursing and social work discharge services, consultation to home care agencies and nursing homes, and health education to the community (Ruster, 1995), spanning the hierarchy of primary, secondary, and tertiary care levels.

A nationwide study of hospital social work reported in Berger and colleagues (1996) revealed that hospitals in the United States today have diversified: while 89 percent of those reporting offer both acute and ambulatory services, 48 percent also offer subacute or extended care; 62 percent, home care; 36 percent, durable medical equipment; and 29 percent, home infusion services (1996:168). Such vertical integration of the continuum of health care services may raise issues concerning free-market competition to achieve cost control (Robinson, 1994:265).

Horizontal Integration Within Hospital Organizations

There also is a trend toward hospitals in the United States moving from bureaucratically structured ones, with a hierarchial chain of command across various levels of management, to a new model of a "horizontally integrative" organization, with a flattening of administrative structure, involving a reduction in middle management and professional group boundaries across functions and organizational units. The objective is an increase in cost-effectiveness through collaboration, coordination, and shared resources (Globerman and Bogo, 1995). In such a horizontally integrative organization, an interdisciplinary work group is organized around a level of care, such as trauma, or a client category, such as aging, and its management is referred to as the "program management" (5).

Globerman and Bogo (1995) argue that such an integrative organization is more compatible with social work values than a bureaucratic one, but does raise the question of how a particular professional group will retain its identity and standards in this atmosphere. Globerman, Davies, and Walsh (1996) report that while hospital social workers surveyed in Ontario, Canada, express concerns about the effect of the new integrative organizational model on control over the nature of their work and role, and on changes in whom they report to, they also felt it is important for hospital social workers to develop understanding of the new types of organizational structures, in terms of their theory, rationale, and positive potential (182).

Elsewhere in the literature, a hospital social work director has described her participation in a leadership training program that taught her how to engage all the staff in "brainstorming" solutions to department problems. This allows on-line staff to replace the traditional middle manager role so that participatory democracy becomes a reality, compatible with the integrative organizational concept (Mayer, 1995).

Impact of Organizational Changes on Hospital Social Work

The percentage of free-standing hospitals, which was 62.5 percent in 1992, dropped to 45.2 percent by 1994, with a commensurate increase in multihospital systems. While most of the reporting hospitals continued in 1994 to have a centralized social work department, there was some increase in decentralized social work services. In addition, there appeared to be some decrease in "middle management," and 21 percent of social work departments had merged with a non-social work department. Nearly one-third had experienced formal reviews by management of, for example, staffing and productivity. While most (77.5 percent) hospitals still had MSW social work managers or directors, many reported some increase in nursing staff in social work departments. Most hospitals also reported similar changes occurring in other areas of the organization. Some decrease in social work responsibility for discharge planning was also reported. Overall, most reports did not regard the changes as negative (Berger et al., 1996:172-173).

In this age of the spread of profit-making hospitals, the issue may be raised as to the comparative costs and quality of services of for-profit vis à vis nonprofit hospitals. Ortiz and Bassoff (1988) reported that for-profit hospitals employ a significantly lower percentage of social work directors who belong to the social work in health care major professional organization, the Society for Social Work Leadership in Health Care. Furthermore, none of the proprietary hospitals were university affiliated and were more likely to be in urban than rural areas. Far fewer hospital social work directors had degrees in social work, and they generally had lower levels of formal education. The authors concluded that the same array of social services was offered by both for-profit and nonprofit hospital social work staff, but were provided by persons with less education in the for-profit organizations.

CLIENT PROBLEMS
AND SOCIAL WORKER FUNCTIONS

Client Problems

The NASW (1990) has categorized the major problems of hospital patients and their families addressed by hospital social workers as including the following:

- Problems related to care and activities of daily living
- Environmental problems
- Patient and family adverse reactions or dysfunctional adjustment to illness and changes in functional status
- Problems related to physical, sexual, and emotional maltreatment

- Relationship problems
- Problems of behavior and cognition and mental disorders, including substance abuse
- Vocational and educational problems
- Legal problems (NASW, 1990:4-5)

Social Worker Functions

The hospital social worker role has evolved over time, resulting in a wide range of expectations for the position (Caputi, 1978). This fact, coupled with the traditional division between medical and psychiatric social work in hospitals, combined with a long history of lack of agreement between social workers and physicians and nurses concerning role expectations for hospital social workers, tends to produce a lack of a clearly defined professional identity (Germain, 1980).

According to the American Hospital Association Profile of United States Hospitals (American Hospital Association, 1993/1994) "organized social work services" means

> Services that are properly directed and sufficiently staffed by qualified individuals who provide assistance and counseling to patients and their families in dealing with social, emotional, and environmental problems associated with illness or disability, often in the context of financial or discharge planning coordination. (xxviii)

The *Health Care Financing Administration* (HCFA) of the federal government, which administers Medicare and Medicaid and establishes the *conditions of participation* (COP) in these government financing programs, currently defines *qualified social worker* as a person with an MSW degree or its equivalent from a social work educational program accredited by the Council on Social Work Education; the HCFA defines a *social work assistant* as a person with a bachelor's degree in social work or a related field who is supervised by a person with an MSW (NASW, 1997).

The *principle* of social work in health care in general has been articulated by NASW as follows:

Social work services shall be an integral part of every health care organization. The services shall be provided to individuals, their families and significant others; to special population groups; to communities; and to special health-related programs, and educational systems.

To provide comprehensiveness and continuity of care, social work services shall encompass the following:

1. The promotion and maintenance of physical and psychosocial well-being.
2. The promotion of conditions essential to assure maximum benefits from short and long-term care services.
3. The prevention of physical or mental illness.
4. The promotion and enhancement of physical and psychosocial functioning, with attention to the social and emotional impact of illness or disability.
5. The promotion of ethical responses to address the often conflicting value positions held by various parties involved in health care settings. (1987:3)

NASW has also developed *clinical indicators* for social work services in the acute care medical hospital, which include the following:

1. *Case finding and access:* that patients needing social work services receive them
2. *Discharge delays:* that the amount of care received is not excessive
3. *Patient and family involvement in planning:* that social workers involve patients and families in making their own decisions about posthospital care
4. *Timeliness:* that patients receive social work services early in the hospitalization
5. *Teamwork:* that patient discharge occurs with the knowledge of the social worker coordinating discharge planning (1990:6)

Case Finding

For many years, hospital social workers depended largely on referrals from physicians and nurses for identification of patients needing social work services. However, as early as 1977, the American Hospital Association published indicators of *high social risk* in acute-care hospitals as a tool for professional standards review for hospital social work (American Hospital Association, 1977). Although, currently, the indicators used vary somewhat among hospitals, in many hospitals today, patients are identified and automatically referred to hospital social work if the patient characteristics include any of the following: age sixty-five or over and living alone; terminal or chronic illness, disability, disfigurement, or accidental injuries; suicidal tendencies; mental retardation or mental health problem; unusually passive or aggressive behavior; health problem-induced employment limitations; low-income, unwed, minor mother (Becker and Becker, 1986:27); and lack of social supports (Berkman et al., 1991). Such screening may be done at admission or prior to admission (Coulton, 1988).

Coulton (1988) pointed out that the ideal screening mechanism rates high on both sensitivity and specificity. *Sensitivity* refers to the ability of the process to identify people needing help with discharge planning and is referred to in research as "target effectiveness," whereas *specificity* is the ability of the screening mechanism to exclude persons who do not need help with discharge planning, what research methodology calls "target efficiency." In other words, a good high-social-risk screening system in a hospital will identify a high percentage of persons of the type the system intended to identify and will not falsely identify many of those which the system did not intend to pick up.

Wolock and colleagues (1987) found that screening tools current at that time needed to be refined to improve both sensitivity and specificity.

Evans and Connis (1996) developed a simple index for VA hospital social worker use as a tool in screening for high risk of placement, death, or readmission—and therefore of need for early social work intervention—and determined that, of the variables they included, the ones that best predicted outcome were *comorbidity* (more than one health problem), mental status, living arrangement, prior institutional admission, prior hospital admission, *iatrogenic* (secondary to treatment) trauma, and pending litigation. However, they admitted that their tool rated highly on sensitivity but low on specificity.

In spite of the increase in high-risk screening, nearly one-half of hospital social work cases still may be referred by non-social workers. One large study of elderly posthospital patients found that 26 percent were identified by the social workers through screening admission summaries, and another 20 percent were picked up through social workers making rounds with other professional staff, while nearly one-half (49 percent) had been referred to social work by another type of health care professional (Oktay et al., 1992:294).

Pray (1991:184) has noted that hospitals vary in the extent to which the social workers are dependent on physicians for referrals (a *closed referral system*) as compared with a system that allows anyone to refer to the hospital social workers (an *open referral system*). However, even in open referral systems, the physician can influence referrals by others to the social workers by interpreting the social worker role to patients and families, as the physician understands (or misunderstands) it (185).

Pray (1991) found variation in perceptions among physicians of what appropriate referrals to hospital social workers include. Still, Pray (1991), similar to Cowles and Lefcowitz (1995), found that physicians were far more likely to refer patients to hospital social workers for concrete-instrumental or social environmental problems, such as those involving financial needs, posthospital care, and transportation, than for primarily affective-expressive problems revolving around attitudes, feelings, or behaviors related to health.

Discharge Planning

Assisting patients with timely arrangements for their posthospital care continues to be a central function of social workers in many hospitals, especially since the 1984 onset of the *prospective payment system* (PPS), according to which hospitals are reimbursed by Medicare in a preset amount based on the estimated number of inpatient days required, given the particular diagnosis and planned procedure, that is, diagnosis-related group (DRG).

In spite of the increased pressure for rapid discharge, Resnick and Dziegielewski (1996) report, from their 1993 survey of hospital social workers and others doing discharge planning, that most claim satisfaction with their work and with client termination and outcome.

Furthermore, Stuen and Monk (1990) conducted a survey of 141 patients discharged from three acute-care hospitals in New York City and found that most patients were satisfied with their inpatient care, the discharge plan, and the posthospital care they received. However, among those who were not satisfied, a significantly higher percentage had chronic health conditions. Stuen and Monk speculate that the reason for this finding may be that the hospitals and home health care programs tend to be geared to acute care more than the ongoing functional limitations of persons with chronic health conditions (1990:16).

On the other hand, Clemens (1995) conducted a study in one teaching hospital with a high percentage of elderly patients of a variety of ethnic backgrounds, for most of whom English was their second language. Clemens found that although the social workers perceived that they had done a good job with the discharge planning of the forty randomly selected cases, the family caregivers presented quite a different interpretation, with many perceiving that the wishes of neither themselves nor the patients had been sufficiently heeded. Apparently, in this teaching hospital, the physicians decided within twenty-four hours whether patients were candidates for home care or nursing home care and referred them to one of two discharge planning departments, one staffed by nurses, the other by social workers, depending on the physicians' judgment. As a result, once the referral was made, the final decision tended to be a foregone conclusion.

This study reveals an example of how the organizational structure of the hospital itself can significantly influence the process followed by departmental staff, with implications for professional autonomy and ethics. Worse yet, the family caregivers felt that their ethnicity had been responded to with a lack of sensitivity by discharge planners, and the discharge planning staff admitted they tended to make less effort to engage family caregivers when they presupposed there might be a language barrier, even though the hospital had foreign language interpreters available (Clemens, 1995:259).

The Bartlett and Baum (1995) follow-up study of hospital patients discharged by hospital social workers to nursing homes underscores the importance of social workers evaluating their practice and provides a brief interview guide to use in follow-up phone interviews to assess discharge outcomes. They found that of 136 patients followed up, 28 percent were still in the nursing home, 23 percent had died, 21 percent were readmitted to the hospital, 12 percent were excluded for reasons of missing data or unusable data, 10 percent had been discharged from the nursing home, and 6 percent were transferred elsewhere (75).

Still another study (Travis, Moore, and McAuley, 1991) examined the social work records of 480 discharged patients and found that 84 percent of the total returned home after discharge, 11.5 percent went to institutional placements, and the remainder died before they could be discharged.

In addition, all social workers who work with psychiatric patients with chronic mental illness need to become aware of the difficulties often faced by the families of these patients and to take appropriate steps to try to correct the reported problems. For example, a qualitative study of thirty-four such families found that most felt they were not provided with enough information by the hospital prior to discharge of patients to their care, that there was a lack of follow-up by the hospital or mental health center, a lack of immediate service available when needed, and a lack of help in getting the patient to follow through with referrals to outpatient community services (Hanson and Rapp, 1992). The families' overall complaints suggest that hospitals are perceived as "dumping on families" through their discharge-planning procedures; this resembles some other study findings reported in this chapter of family members' perceptions of elderly patients concerning the discharge-planning process.

The challenge of discharge planning. Many patients are considered "ready for discharge" and accordingly referred to hospital social workers and other discharge planners even though one or more of the following conditions exist:

- The patient may be insufficiently recovered from the acute health condition to take care of himself or herself.
- The patient may be mentally confused, emotionally depressed, or otherwise mentally impaired, permanently or temporarily.
- The patient may need oxygen, an in-dwelling catheter that requires irrigating and changing, assistance with eating, dressing, walking, bathing, toileting, and so forth.

- The patient may have a new baby with special problems, but has never cared for an infant before.
- The patient now has a seizure disorder and his or her family has never seen a grand mal seizure before.
- The patient has been advised not to climb stairs, but lives in a second-floor apartment with no elevator access.
- The patient has AIDS and the family has not yet been informed.
- The patient is a young man, now permanently paralyzed from the waist down, and his only family lives in a rural mountain area several hundred miles away.
- The patient is a young mother with several children to care for, but she will be unable to do any lifting for several weeks and the father is undependable.
- The patient will need to return to the hospital twice a week for an indefinite period of time for kidney dialysis treatments and he or she has no personal transportation.

These are some examples of "the challenge of discharge planning" for the social worker or whoever else is assigned the responsibility. It should be evident from these examples that discharge planning requires much more than simply referring the client to a nursing home or home health care agency. The kinds of services often involved in hospital discharge planning include assessment, referrals, planning and coordination, family education, patient education, patient counseling, postdischarge follow-up, and family counseling (Oktay et al., 1992:294).

Abramson and colleagues (1993) have concluded from their study of the level of disagreement among the various interested parties in discharge-planning situations that a high level of disagreement is not unusual, but rather the norm. This indicates the need for clinical social worker skills in discharge planning to effectively elicit and explore the participants' perspectives and to achieve equitable conflict resolution (62).

Another study (Proctor et al., 1995) of pediatric discharge planning reported that their results also indicate the complexity of the discharge-planning process, which is influenced by family, resources, and teamwork. Nearly all (90 percent) of the 105 cases involved one or more complications, the most common (67 percent) being financial or lack of economic resources to obtain the needed services, largely reflecting the fact that at least thirty million American children have no health insurance, and one-fourth of all children in America live in families with incomes below the official government poverty line (Proctor et al., 1995:9, 15).

The significance of quality discharge planning to cost savings is indicated by study findings that the earlier the hospital social worker intervention with a patient, the shorter the patient's length of stay (Evans et al., 1989:277; Fillit et al., 1992).

A study (Soskolne and Auslander, 1993) conducted in Israel examined the comparative effect on patient posthospital care services of implementing *discharge-planning protocol training* of hospital social workers. The study found that a significantly higher percentage of patients in the group whose social workers participated in the departmental training program in discharge planning not only received formal home health care services but received them for a longer period of time than the patients served by the social workers before their discharge-planning training.

The importance of interdisciplinary collaboration is underscored by the findings of a study by Feather (1993) of discharge planners from a random sample of all U.S. hospitals to determine their perceptions of the variables determining effective discharge planning. Feather (1993) found that the single most important factor is "cooperation and support from the physician staff of the hospital" (1). Later, Feather commented, "if discharge planners have power and clarity, almost any model of discharge planning can be effective, whether the hospital is large or small, rural or urban" (11). Feather suggests that hospital discharge planners focus more on strategies to enhance the understanding and cooperation of physicians and other hospital personnel concerning the discharge—planning function (12).

The Need for Improved Patient and Family Involvement in Decision Making

Coulton (1990) has reviewed the research relating to patient and family involvement in decision making. Her concerns are as follows:

- Patients and families do not always understand what their options are and the implications of each.
- Patients and families may have difficulty focusing on the issues at hand because of anxiety about the health condition.
- Patients and families often have so little time to make important decisions concerning life-sustaining measures or posthospital care that they are unable to think them through adequately.
- Hospital records sometimes indicate a patient's choice about serious matters such as whether or not to resuscitate, with little or no documentation of patient or family involvement in the decision making.
- Several studies have found lack of agreement between the physician, social worker, patient, and family concerning perceptions of the patient's position on such issues.
- There is some evidence that a patient's decisions may be "led" so that it is questionable whether what is recorded is actually what the patient wants.
- A major problem suggested by study findings on patient and family involvement in decision making is whether their assumptions were accurate, that is, whether they fully understood both the pros and cons of each alternative.
- There also is some evidence that patients prefer a family member they trust to make decisions over their physician.
- The outcome for most patients improves the more they perceive that they were adequately involved in decision making concerning themselves.

Elsewhere, Coulton and colleagues (1989) reported that among patients with an *internal locus of control*, posthospital anxiety decreases with an increase in perceived control over the discharge plan.

Abramson (1990), too, has expressed concern about the danger of compromising the social work value of client self-determination and of the primacy of client interests; she reviews the evidence of the importance of feeling in control to well-being, health status, and even survival (54-55). Abramson recommends the social worker offer choices to clients and explore rather than ignore signs of conflict between the key participants, continually advocating for the patients' right to control over decision making concerning their own lives (56).

Advocacy in Hospital Social Work

One Canadian study (Herbert and Levin, 1996) of hospital social workers' perceptions of their own role, including advocacy, found that they reportedly spend the least amount of time on advocacy, compared with assessment, counseling, resource linkage, and consultation/collaboration (71). The same finding was obtained by Oktay and colleagues in a study of Baltimore hospital social work (1992:294). Canadian hospitals are undergoing a similar reorganization process as U.S. hospitals, with similar effects on their social workers. The general consensus among social workers seems to be "don't make waves," which reflects a general sense of disempowerment (Herbert and Levin, 1996:82).

However, Dobrof (1991) commented on the findings of past research on the impact of the DRG system that "It is imperative that the social work profession use its expert advocacy skills to promote both an increase in post-hospital health care resources and to develop mechanisms for financing this care" (50).

Critical Incident Stress Debriefing (CISD)

In efforts to survive hospital reorganization, downsizing, and demands for evidence of value, some hospital social work departments have found inventive ways to demonstrate their importance to the hospital system. One example of this is described by Spitzer and Neely (1992) and Spitzer and Burke (1993), who played a leadership role in developing a statewide system in Oregon for providing *debriefing* services to providers of emergency services in crisis situations.

The premise is that service providers such as police, firefighters, and emergency medical technicians, as well as emergency room personnel, often suffer personal trauma from their battlefield-like experiences, and need help to release their subsequent feelings, which otherwise can accumulate and cause harm to themselves and others in the form of such reactions as depression, violence, and physical illness.

Spitzer and Neely (1992) describe the six stages in the debriefing process, which lasts about three hours. This is an excellent article that should be read by anyone interested in learning more about how to develop such a stress-debriefing service, which its authors report brought state and national recognition to their hospital social work department and "united local fire, ambulance, clergy, mental health and medical professionals into one of the largest critical stress debriefing teams in the U.S." (56).

Crisis Intervention in the Emergency Room

In 1996, the Task Force on Adolescent Assault Victim Needs of the American Academy of Pediatrics published a model protocol for providers of hospital-based pediatric emergency and trauma care, out of concern for the increase in adolescent victims of violent assault being seen in hospital emergency departments, often attended by personnel with a lack of understanding of how to deal with the psychosocial aspects of such situations. The protocol includes specific steps for social workers, pediatric psychologists, and psychiatrists to follow, such as critical incident stress debriefing (CISD) for the victim and family, if needed; evaluating the circumstances of the assault; evaluating the victim's psychological functioning before the injury and his or her response to the incident; arranging for follow-up mental health services, if needed; assisting the family with discharge planning (which may include a change of residence and/or schools); ongoing supportive assistance to the victim and family if they are required to identify the assailant or testify in court; and periodic postdischarge assessment of victim and family follow-through with needed services and of the status of possible post-traumatic stress syndrome (Task Force on Adolescent Assault Victim Needs, 1996:998).

Bloch (1996) has written about her experience as chief of clinical social work services in the emergency department of a large urban medical center in terms of how the social worker can help family members when the patient is critically ill or injured, likely to die, and does die in the emergency room. Bloch (1996) stresses the importance of providing such families with a special room in which to wait, of keeping them informed of medical efforts and the patient status and interpreting the condition to them, and of the social worker remaining when the physician enters and provides a brief review of what has happened, concluding with a simple but gentle statement informing the family of the death. Bloch (1996) also shares what she has learned from experience about such issues as the family viewing the body, initiating discussion of organ and tissue donation, a coroner exam or autopsy by the hospital, the funeral arrangements, and care of the closest or most distressed family survivor.

Other common social work services in hospital emergency departments include brief counseling and referral and resource finding for patients and families with such presenting problems as attempted or threatened suicide, child abuse, domestic violence, chemical dependency, acute psychiatric problem behavior, rape, assault and battery, and homelessness. Such social work services can be cost-effective for the hospital (Ponto and Berg, 1992) and more effective for the patients, who otherwise tend to keep coming back because, without social work intervention in such cases, the underlying psychosocial problems often are not addressed by medical personnel (Keehn, Roglitz, and Bowden, 1994).

Another group of people who tend to use hospital emergency department medical services inappropriately, who can be more effectively and efficiently helped by social workers instead, consists of certain elderly people who tend to seek help for physical complaints when the problem is a mental health one and those with chronic health problems in acute episodes because of noncompliance associated with psychosocial problems (McCoy, Kipp, and Ahern, 1992). Such social work intervention can reduce repeat utilization of this sort.

Hospital emergency departments are excellent places for social work students to obtain training in the assessment, treatment, and disposition of patients with psychiatric problems (Walsh, 1985).

Other Hospital Social Worker Functions

Elder abuse. Of course, many patients with psychosocial problems who are first seen in the emergency room are subsequently admitted to inpatient care and seen by social workers assigned to special medical or surgical units, as a result of referrals to social work or of high-risk screening systems. Elder abuse is another such problem that may be increasing, as a result, perhaps, of both the growth of the elderly population and the shortened hospital stays and increased burden on family members to provide personal care services to sometimes severely impaired family members. Such situations are an example of the need for collaboration between the medical and social work staff of hospitals (Hazard, 1995).

Child sexual abuse. Child sexual abuse is another psychosocial problem that is sometimes identified among pediatric patients in hospitals. Dubowitz, Black, and Harrington (1992) reported on the findings of a study to determine which types of evidence collected by an interdisciplinary team, including a pediatrician, child psychologist, and pediatric social worker, best helped to diagnose child sexual abuse. The results indicated that the child's disclosure of having been sexually abused and positive physical examination findings most influenced team members' conclusion, whereas sexualized behavior of the child, somatic problems, and the child's response to the physical exam did not contribute (688), as these may be indicative of life experiences other than sexual abuse. In this study,

> The [hospital] social worker assessment included a history of the alleged abuse, the family's response to the allegation, the involvement of public agencies, and sources of support to the family. In addition, the social worker assessed the functioning of the family, parental concerns regarding the child, and access to services. (1992:689)

KNOWLEDGE REQUIREMENTS

Specific Client Populations and Problems

Hospital social workers need knowledge concerning the medical and social implications of specific health conditions, in terms of their prognosis and treatment and probable psychosocial problems, appropriate resources to address the needs, and information about how to access them (Rauch and Schreiber, 1985:215; Ross, 1993:244-245).

Fahs and Wade (1996) found that AIDS patients are significantly benefited by being hospitalized in specialized units with an interdisciplinary team having expertise regarding this health condition. This team should include a social worker with specialized knowledge and skills who can facilitate discharge planning through knowledge of specialized resources (29). Furthermore, Beckerman and Rock (1996), through a survey of hospital social workers who specialize in working with AIDS patients, found that some common themes emerge from their experience, pointing both to the challenges and rewards of their work. One of the reported rewards is that the interdisciplinary team tends to become more mutually supportive and cooperative than usual in hospitals, apparently as a result of the emotional intensity of the shared experience (86).

The hospital social worker also needs to have knowledge of "response patterns of particular ethnic and cultural groups and be able to intervene with them appropriately" (Ross, 1995:1373).

The Organizational Setting

In addition, hospital social workers need to understand the cultures, roles, and functions of other professionals in the setting and how to work collaboratively with them; they must have mastery of the vocabulary of the health care world and know the community resources for various types of health problems and how to access them (Rauch and Schreiber, 1985:215).

Community Resources

Having knowledge of community resources is more than knowing which resources exist for which particular need; it is also important to develop and continually strive to update more intimate knowledge of the quality of such resources, such as nursing homes, home care agencies, and medical aids and appliances providers. Hospital social workers who link clients with such resources need to visit these places (Dobrof, 1991:51), get to know the people who work in them, and do follow-up studies of referred clients. Such studies should include asking patients and family members their opinions on the quality of the services they received, in terms of timeliness, interpersonal treatment, the condition of physical equipment, and the competence of the personnel.

Intervention Modalities

Since discharge planning is often central to the hospital social worker role, it is essential that hospital social workers understand what is involved in effective and efficient discharge planning and recognize that it is not simply a "concrete service," but one requiring considerable clinical skill (Donnelly, 1992:108). Rauch and Schreiber (1985) present a framework for training in discharge planning that is directed toward demonstrating its clinical aspects.

Needed Research, Evaluation, and Documentation

Ross (1995) argues that hospital social workers need to have a sufficient grasp of existing knowledge in a particular area to plan and conduct research for knowledge development (1373-1374).

As has been noted elsewhere in this book, the current focal interests in the field of health services research are *outcomes and effectiveness* (Marcus, 1990). That is, cost-effectiveness continues to be "the name of the game," and social work research in health care needs to continue to improve its management information systems, which are essential sources of research data, and also continue to improve its research quality, attending especially to issues of external validity and instrument reliability (84).

Hospital social workers must learn what is required of them in terms of documentation of their work for use by other health professionals in the setting, for Medicare and Medicaid reimbursement purposes, and for quality assurance and peer review purposes.

Practice Experience in Knowledge Development

Ideally, perhaps, future hospital social workers should have a field placement in a hospital in order to enhance their experience and desire to remain in hospital social work. Showers (1992) found five areas of field practicum in which students' satisfaction with their field placement was most predictive: (1) satisfaction with the supervisory relationship was most predictive of satisfaction with the field instructor; (2) supervisory teaching was most predictive of satisfaction with the learning experience; (3) variety of opportunities was most predictive of satisfaction with the program; (4) stress level was most predictive of satisfaction with the hospital; and (5) the level of field program organization and coordination between field instructors was found most predictive of the overall fieldwork experience (31).

In relation to the third area identified, another study (Cuzzi et al., 1996) also found that social work students who experienced three rotations during their hospital field placement reported greater satisfaction with their experience than a control group of social work students who remained on the same medical or surgical service throughout their placement. Cuzzi and colleagues (1996) attribute this finding to the fact that hospital social workers today have more diverse caseloads and the profession needs "expert generic social work practitioners" (76).

The University of Iowa School of Social Work has developed an innovative approach to teaching practice research skills to MSW students in an advanced research methods course. It involves giving students the option of doing a "research practicum" at a local medical center where they would work closely with a social work practitioner in health care. The union of student and practitioner proved productive for both, as the practitioner could identify issues for practice research while the student had the research skills to design an appropriate study (Hall et al., 1996).

VALUES AND ETHICS CONSIDERATIONS

Foster and colleagues (1993) surveyed 255 hospital social workers concerning how they deal with certain ethical dilemmas in practice and what they perceive as their needs for training in bioethics. They found that most social workers felt well prepared to deal with ethical issues in practice situations, but still expressed a desire for more training, particularly concerning the rationing of health care.

Foster and colleagues (1993) note that while rationing of health care is associated with such issues as who will and will not receive organ transplants and other high-cost procedures, such rationing is, in fact, involved in social work high-risk screening and discharge planning in the sense that the process of selecting certain patients for service implies an exclusion of others. In addition, discharge-planning decisions clearly involve rationing, as determined by reimbursement policies of public and private health insurance as well as out-of-pocket financial resources of clients. For example, Morrow-Howell and Proctor (1994), in their study of the determinants of hospital discharge-planning destination, reported that patients with Medicaid coverage were eleven times more likely to be discharged to a nursing home (493).

Abramson (1996) explores four alternative approaches to ethical understanding in social work, which she labels the (1) principles approach, (2) virtue ethics, (3) feminist ethics, and (4) Afrocentricity. Abramson (1996) presents the "principles approach" as rooted in the false notion that there is consensus about the relative importance of underlying values or principles that can be discerned dispassionately. In comparison, "virtue ethics" revolves around efforts to discern and weigh the underlying motivations of the players. "Feminist ethics," the third approach, takes a variety of forms revolving around combating oppression at both the micro and macro levels. Finally, "Afrocentricity" is depicted as reflecting concern for the well-being of the family and community and for past and future generations, as well as respect for human feelings and dignity.

Abramson (1996) reminds us that an emerging trend today is to have a more flexible and receptive attitude toward alternative *paradigms* (worldviews). This can serve to enrich and sensitize health care social workers' capacity for relatedness to diverse human dilemmas in today's health care environment, which can be fraught with glib rationalizations for unethical actions.

Judith Ross (1993) asked, "it is imperative that a social work presence in health be sustained, but if it means relinquishing our commitment to the profession and to social work values, principles, and goals, is the expense too great?" (244).

Dobrof (1991) also has expressed concern about the possible negative impact of the DRG system on the role and satisfaction of the hospital social worker and on the well-being of the discharged patient and his or her family, whose right to "self-determination" may be seriously compromised by the pressures of cost containment (46).

Although the Clemens (1995) study discussed earlier under Discharge Planning is only one small study, which may in no way be considered representative, the fact that the reported findings occur at all supports concern that professional social work ethics are at risk in hospital practice.

SKILL REQUIREMENTS

Bennett, Legon, and Zilberfein (1989) have suggested that hospital social workers try to counteract the potentially negative effects of "aggressive" discharge planning by exercising greater "empathy" with clients. They regard this as a skill that can be developed with supervisor assistance in heightening worker self-awareness and understanding of the client's position concerning discharge-planning preferences.

However, consideration should perhaps be given to the possibility that a profession may be better off not to continue in certain settings when conditions there prevent them from practicing in accordance with their professional knowledge and/or their professional values and ethics.

Even if social work does not survive in hospital settings, it may well be that it could be more appropriately utilized elsewhere in health care. For example, Ross (1993) proposed that as hospitals reduce length of stay and inpatient acute care, they will increasingly compete for survival with providers of other levels of care, such as primary care and prevention, where social work may fit very well:

> Relationship building and counseling and communication skills that are integral to our work should be appreciated in primary care and health prevention and could contribute to developing consumer-oriented strategies beyond the current conception and practice as competition for patients intensifies. Understanding of and ability to negotiate systems will help position social workers to assume new roles and new assignments. (Ross, 1993:246)

HELPING INTERVENTIONS

Among the many available interventions for social workers to use in their work in hospitals are screening and case finding, crisis intervention, psychosocial assessment and intervention planning, brief counseling, bereavement services, discharge planning, post-discharge follow-up and outreach, group work, emergency services through on-call programs, documentation and record keeping, and collaboration (Ross, 1995).

Group Work

In addition to those interventions discussed earlier in the section Social Worker Functions, Glassman (1991) reminds us of the varied uses of social group work in health care settings and of its special healing potential, such as self-help, mutual support, education, coping with crises, self-esteem and empowerment building, family and significant other support development, as well as a medium for interdisciplinary teamwork through coleadership or rotating leadership of group sessions.

Hanson and colleagues (1994) found that hospital inpatients being treated for alcoholism were significantly more likely to follow through with outpatient support group participation and to have lower rates of recidivism if they began their participation in such a support group with other recovering alcoholics prior to hospital discharge, thereby facilitating the transition from inpatient to outpatient status.

Innovative Interventions

Gentry (1993) has reported on an innovative service provided by a hospital in Philadelphia. The service came about as a result of a growing problem of "boarder babies," or newborns in fragile health as a result of prematurity and/or alcohol and drug absorption in utero. The babies' parents are generally unable or unwilling to assume responsibility for their care so they remain in the hospital for a prolonged period of time. When the local child placement agencies were unable to rapidly find foster homes for the infants, hospital employees began to inquire about whether they might serve as foster parents. The social work department discovered that it was able to expedite the placement process by providing an "information and referral" service to the employees concerning the procedure for applying to become a certified foster parent (Gentry, 1993).

COMMENTARY

One cannot read the hospital social work literature today without sensing a sort of desperation and determination to do "whatever it takes to hold on."

As suggested by Ross (1993), the profession needs to examine the alternative to continued practice in some of the current settings of social work in health care and seek the path that places what we know is right above what it takes for mere survival.

Chapter 5

Social Work
in Home Health Care/Home Care

HISTORICAL BACKGROUND

The Concept of Home Care

The term *home care* is used here as an umbrella concept to include both home health services that provide skilled services, such as nursing, physical therapy, and speech therapy, and the so-called "unskilled" services, such as homemaker and chore services and personal care services, that provide assistance with *activities of daily living* (ADLs). As the NASW Standards for Social Work in Health Care Settings state:

> Thus home care cannot be viewed as only medical service. Home health care includes an array of services—nursing, rehabilitative therapies, social work, personal care, homemaking—to aid the individual in achieving and sustaining the highest level of health, activity, and independence. (NASW, 1987:27)

In the literature, the terms home health care (HHC) and home care are sometimes used interchangeably, sometimes to refer to distinct types of services, and sometimes to refer to home health care as a subdivision of home care, the use employed here.

The Growth and Development of Home Care

The home was the original location of most health care, which was provided by family, friends, and neighbors with the support and supervision of a physician who visited occasionally.

Beginning in the latter half of the 1800s, voluntary, nonprofit agencies, such as visiting nurse organizations, began to provide *formal home care services* (i.e., other than family or friend provided) in the form of maternal and child care (Balinsky, 1994:1).

The concept of home-visiting nurses emerged in the mid-1800s and was the forerunner of public health nursing, now called community health nursing, and preceded what we now call home health care (Clemen-Stone, Eigsti, and McGuire, 1987:8). The first Visiting Nurse Association was organized in Buffalo, New York, in 1885, and many others soon emerged around the United States and continue today to be significant providers of home health care (158), especially in urban areas—14 percent in urban areas and 5 percent in rural areas (Kenney, 1993).

Public health nursing has its roots in the early work of a leader in the history of nursing (and social work), Lillian D. Wald, who founded the Henry Street Settlement House in New York City in 1893 (Clemen-Stone, Eigsti, and McGuire, 1987:9-10). However, the concept of public health nursing originally was not associated with government funding or service, but only later was gradually adopted by city, state, and finally the federal government as, appropriately, a public tax-supported service (14-15).

Public health nursing, as well as social work, emerged in response to the multiple social and health problems of the latter half of the 1800s that accompanied industrialization, urbanization, and immigration in America. Infant and maternal mortality and contagious and infectious disease were rampant as a result of the social changes of the period (Clemen-Stone, Eigsti, and McGuire, 1987:14).

Historically, while private, nonprofit nursing agencies could provide hands-on care, such as changing dressings and catheters and bathing patients, the public health nurses were legally required to confine their interventions to supervision, instruction, and monitoring communicable disease functions. Today, both types of agencies provide hands-on care through their home health care services.

Around the beginning of the twentieth century, the seat of health care shifted from home to the hospital (Cannon, 1923). Now, as we enter the twenty-first century, the trend is toward moving health care back to the home and community (Balinsky, 1994:1; Simmons, 1994). In 1955, the U.S. Public Health Service endorsed the physician-oriented home care program, designed to provide medical and social services to patients at home through a professional group minimally composed of a physician, nurse, and social worker (NASW, 1987:27).

The Growth of the Proprietary Sector in Home Care

Until the latter half of the 1960s, formal home health care services were largely provided by nonprofit organizations, such as the Visiting Nurse Association, and public agencies, such as the Public Health Departments. After Title XVIII (Medicare) and Title XIX (Medicaid) were enacted by Congress in 1965, proprietary (for-profit) home care programs "mushroomed." Although the first hospital-based home care service was established in New York City in 1947 at Montefiore Hospital (Balinsky, 1994:1; Blazer, 1988), as of 1967, there were only 133 hospital-based home care agencies and no proprietary freestanding home care agencies (Balinsky, 1994:2). However, by 1997, freestanding proprietary agencies comprised nearly one-half (47 percent) and hospital-based agencies constituted more than one-fourth (26 percent) of all certified HHC agencies (National Association for Home Care, 1997).

Home health care has proved to be one of the lucrative human service alternatives to the reduction of manufacturing in the United States (Karger and Stoesz, 1994:227). Part A of Medicare includes coverage for home health care services under medical supervision, provided that (1) the patient requires *skilled* care (professional nursing services, physical therapy, or speech therapy), (2) the patient is essentially homebound, and (3) the physician certifies that conditions (1) and (2) do exist (Balinsky, 1994:3).

In 1994, for-profit home health care organizations had combined annual receipts/revenue of $14.916 billion, while nonprofit HHC organizations had $7.944 billion in annual receipts/revenue, only slightly more than one-half (53.3 percent) of for-profit HHC organization income (U.S. Government Printing Office, 1995b:122). During 1994, proprietary HHC agencies constituted 43.8 percent of all such agencies in the United States, and voluntary nonprofit HHC agencies represented 36.8 percent, while the remaining 19.5 percent of HHC agencies were operated by government or "other" (U.S. Government Printing Office, 1995b:135).

Social Work in Home Care

Social work service through Medicare-funded home care is only provided if the physician orders it on the basis of a need directly related to the medical condition (Balinsky, 1994:3). In 1992, the U.S. Department of Labor (DOL) reported that about 26 percent of social workers employed in all "industries" were employed in health services, distributed as shown in Table 5.1, which indicates that slightly less than 1 percent of social workers are employed in home health care services.

Whereas Medicare mandates social worker participation in Medicare-certified hospice programs, in home health care, Medicare only mandates that social work services be available if the physician deems them necessary and medically related, which is largely dependent upon the attending nurse informing the physician of such a need, if perceived.

TABLE 5.1. Percentage Distribution of Social Workers Employed in Home Health Care Relative to Other Settings of Health Service

Hospitals, public and private	14.13
Health and allied services	5.28
Nursing and personal care services	2.99
Offices of physicians	1.48
Offices of other health practitioners	1.22
Home health care services	.90
Medical and dental laboratories	.01
Total percentage of social workers employed in health care settings	26.02

Source: Ginsberg, Leon (1995). *The Social Work Almanac* (Second Edition). Washington, DC: NASW Press, 355. Data obtained from U.S. Department of Labor, Bureau of Labor Statistics, November 1993.

Other Constraints in Home Care Coverage

Home health care through Medicare is not provided twenty-four hours a day. Instead, a family member, friend, or other caregiver must be available. As a result of these restrictions, Medicare only pays for a small part of the home care that exists (Balinsky, 1994:3). Only the very affluent in America who can afford to pay out of pocket for these services receive round-the-clock home health care. Thus, a dual-level system is created, in which the services rendered are determined by individual economic ability rather than need for service (Olson, 1994:30).

The findings of two surveys of home health care agencies conducted in 1986 and 1987 (Binney, Estes, and Ingman, 1990) indicate that medical services had increased most, while social/supportive services were the most commonly requested services they could not provide (761).

Costs and Payers of Home Health Care

Personal health care expenditures in the United States totaled $831.675 billion in 1994. Of the total, approximately $26.158 billion expended in 1994 for HHC, $13.170, or 50 percent, was paid by government programs; $6.101 billion, or 23 percent, was out of pocket; $3.394 billion, or 13 percent, was private health insurance; and the remaining $3.493 billion, or 13 percent, was "other," which includes nonpatient revenues and industrial plants (U.S. Government Printing Office [see Table 5.2], 1995b:115).

Personal health care expenditures combined with costs for administration, construction of medical facilities, and medical research totaled $949.419 billion in 1994.

TABLE 5.2. Home Health Care Expenditures, 1994

$13.170 billion government funded	50%
6.101 billion out of pocket	23%
3.394 billion private health insurance	13%
3.493 billion "other"	13%
$26.158 billion total home health expenditures	100%

Source: U.S. Government Printing Office (1995b). *Statistical Abstracts of the United States.* Washington, DC: Author, 115.

In 1994, Medicare and Medicaid together expended $20.048 billion for HHC services. Medicaid payments for home health services totaled $7.042 billion, or 6.5 percent, of total payments for all Medicaid paid health care services, which equaled $108.270 billion (U.S. Government Printing Office, 1995b:118). During the same year, Medicare expended a total of $13.006 billion, or 7.9 percent of the $164.862 billion total health care paid through Medicare (U.S. Government Printing Office, 1995b:115).

When all sources of payment for home health care services are considered—Medicare, Medicaid, other government programs, private health insurance, and out-of-pocket payments—home health care costs constitute about 3 percent (.0276 percent) of all personal health care expenditures in the United States (U.S. Government Printing Office, 1995b:115).

As of December 1996, the National Association for Home Care (NAHC) had identified a total of 20,215 HHC agencies in the United States and its territories, of which 10,027 (49.6 percent) were Medicare-certified home care agencies; 2,154 were Medicare-certified hospice agencies; and the remaining 8,034 home health, hospice, and home care aide organizations were not Medicare certified and did not participate in Medicare (see Table 5.3) (NAHC, 1997).

Reasons for the Growth of Home Care

Although home health care represents only a small fraction of spending for all personal health care services, about 8 percent of Medicare and 6.5 percent of Medicaid in 1994 (Kaye and Davitt,

TABLE 5.3. Medicare Certification of Home Health Agencies, 1996

10,027	49.6%	Medicare-certified home health care agencies
2,154	10.7%	Medicare-certified hospice care agencies
8,034	39.7%	Non-Medicare-certified home health, hospice or home care aide agencies
20,215	100%	Total home care agencies in the United States

Source: National Association for Home Care (1997). Basic Statistics About Home Care. Washington, DC. NAHC home page: <www.NAHC.org/consumer/hcstats.html>.

1995), it "is the fastest growing segment of the health services industry" in the United States (National Association for Home Care, 1996:9). The reasons for this growth include the following:

1. The aging of the population, especially the *old-old* (people age eighty-five and older) with a high rate of functional disability
2. The shift from acute infectious diseases to *chronic diseases* (incurable but not terminal) as the major health problems
3. Efforts such as the *prospective payment system (PPS)* introduction of *diagnosis-related groups (DRGs)*, initiated in 1983 by Medicare to reduce the use of high-cost hospital services and to reduce the spiraling cost of nursing home care paid for by Medicaid
4. The increase in technology that allows people to be cared for at home in spite of the need for medical equipment such as IVs, catheters, suction machines, portable oxygen, ventilators, and infusion pumps (Balinsky, 1994:9-15; Braus, 1994)
5. The AIDS epidemic (Balinsky, 1994:45-70)
6. The alarming growth of medically fragile children (Balinsky, 1994:23)
7. The lack of economic access to alternative forms of care, such as nursing home care, for many elderly people
8. The poor quality of nursing homes in the United States, which prompts people to choose home care instead (Garner, 1995: 1627; Olson, 1994)
9. By 1993, the transition from using home health care primarily for acute care of posthospitalization cases to using it to care for chronically ill persons (Welch, Wennberg, and Welch, 1996), making the distinction between normal Medicare-covered acute care and long-term care benefits less clear (Kane et al., 1997)

In 1994, Allen J. Goldberg, president-elect of the American Academy of Home Care Physicians, wrote:

Home health care is the next frontier of medical practice and is rapidly being explored for its limitless potential opportunities. . . . Explosive growth has occurred in advance of the definition of public policy, determination of social consensus, and the establishment of a scientific foundation for the state of the art practice. (Goldberg, 1994:911)

THEORETICAL PERSPECTIVES

Although not a clear and developed rationale for home health care, the values and objectives reflected in the U.S. home health care system include (1) cost control through the encouragement of family caregiving; (2) elevation of political concessions to the medical profession and the profit-making business sector over concern for the needs and wishes of patients and families or for issues of social justice and humane caring; and (3) perpetuation of a two-level system of health care, dependent on economic status, that determines the appropriateness of service interventions.

Caring

Ideally, however:

> The objective governing home care is to maximize the independent functioning of the client and the caregiver and to maintain the person in the community. All of the assistance provided is focused on ameliorating problems that impede this functioning. (Cox, 1992:180)

Presumably, home care is preferably for patients of any age, when they want to be at home, and resources are available to adequately provide for their needs there. Most people feel more secure and comfortable at home (Garner, 1995), which, at least theoretically, optimizes their potential sense of well-being and, hence, health status.

Cost Control

In addition, home health care may be less expensive than nursing home care, if family, friends, or neighbors volunteer the basic supportive care services, which are only supplemented by part-time formal home care. As a result, both public and private health insurance programs limit home care to part-time services.

In estimated Medicare charges, the average home care visit cost $88 in 1996, compared with $334 for an average day in a skilled nursing home care facility, or $1,872 for an average day in the hospital (National Association for Home Care, 1996:10).

In 1994, total expenditures for HHC from all sources was $26.158 billion, or 36 percent of total expenditures of $72.253 billion from all sources for nursing home care, and $13.170 billion, or 32 percent of the government's share of nursing home care (U.S. Government Printing Office, 1995b:115).

The Medical Model

Home health care in the United States is a prime example of what has been termed "the medicalization of social problems" (Binney, Estes, and Ingman, 1990).

Although many elderly people do have health problems requiring so-called "skilled care," more simply need supportive assistance for functional impairments, such as difficulty ambulating, dressing, bathing, eating, and taking medications as directed. However, this type of care is not reimbursable by Medicare, either in a nursing home or at home, and is only reimbursable by some state Medicaid waiver programs, if the person is financially indigent (Cox, 1992).

As a result, elderly or disabled people who require such supportive assistance frequently exhaust their personal economic resources in order to become eligible for Medicaid for the very poor. The United States is the only nation in the world for which the leading cause of personal bankruptcy is health care costs (Garner, 1995:1629).

This medicalization of formal home health care services resulted from an effort, when Medicare was introduced to Congress in the mid-1960s, to make the proposed legislation politically palatable to the American Medical Association, which had long resisted any type of government intervention in health care that appeared to threaten the interests of the medical profession. As a result, home health was proposed as only reimbursable through Medicare if it were recommended as "medically necessary" and under physician authorization and supervision. "In sum, Medicare and other health policies for the elderly, e.g., Medicaid, from their origin to the present day, reflect medicine's monopoly in the control and management of the care of the aging" (Binney, Estes, and Ingman, 1990:763-764).

HUMAN DIVERSITY RELEVANCE

Significant differences are found among age groups, gender groups, socioeconomic status groups, ethnic groups, rural/urban groups, and so on, in regard to health behavior, illness behavior, and sick-role behavior, and these diversity variables interact with one another, so that group characteristics are not "additive" (Corin, 1994). In addition, considerable evidence suggests that a sense of empowerment or of being in control plays a significant role in health outcomes (Evans, Barer, and Marmor, 1994), and this seems to be influenced by such things as social supports and being in a culturally integrated, congruent, familiar, and cognitively comfortable environment, one that is rooted in tradition and has status consistency (Corin, 1994).

Therefore, to maximize the potential for positive health outcomes, it behooves social workers in the health field to attend to the clients' attitudes, beliefs, customs, and preferences concerning their health care options, which are often influenced by human diversity.

Ethnicity needs to be a major consideration in social work in home health care, since the nonwhite elderly population is expected to increase markedly. In 1990, 86.7 percent of America's population age sixty-five and over was white, but by 2050, this percentage is expected to decrease to 66.9 (U.S. Department of Health and Human Services, National Institute of Health, National Institute on Aging, 1993). Thus, the nonwhite elderly population is expected to increase from about 13 percent in 1990 to about 33 percent by the year 2050. Table 5.4 depicts these expected changes in the ethnic composition of the U.S. population from 1990 to 2050.

TABLE 5.4. Ethnic Distribution of the U.S. Elderly Population, 1990 and 2050

	1990	2050
White	86.7%	66.9%
Black	7.9	9.6
American Indian	0.3	0.6
Asian	1.4	7.4
Hispanic	3.7	15.5
Total	100.0	100.0

Source: U.S. Department of Health and Human Services, National Institute of Health, National Institute on Aging (1993). *Profiles of America's Elderly: Racial and Ethnic Diversity of America's Elderly Population,* Number 3, November, POP/93-1-8.

Eric Erikson considered cultural identity as essential to achieving "ego integrity":

> For he [the older person] knows that an individual life is the accidental coincidence of but one life cycle with but one segment of history; and that for him all human integrity stands or falls with one style of integrity of which he partakes. (Erikson, 1959:98)

> The style of integrity developed by his culture or civilization thus becomes the patrimony of his soul, the seal of his moral paternity of himself. (Erikson, 1956, cited in Giordano, 1992:24)

Ethnic sensitivity is a manifestation of the social work value of individualizing the client. Since the first step in sensitivity to human diversity is becoming aware of the person's differences, ideally, an "ethnic assessment" ought to be part of the psychosocial assessment in health care situations, including home health care. Fandetti and Goldmeier (1988) provide a framework for such an assessment at the micro, mezzo, and macro levels (see Table 5.5).

Three levels of population and program characteristics interact to determine whether geriatric services are equitably used: *appropriateness* to the health and functional status of the elder; *accessibility* given the social and economic characteristics of the group; and *acceptability* to group-specific norms and expectations (Damon-Rodriguez, Wallace, and Kington, 1994:55).

TABLE 5.5. A Multilevel Ethnic Assessment Framework

Micro: The PERSON
1. Assess the person's cultural orientation: e.g., languages spoken, religion professed, and the generation of immigration of the primary client. 2. Evaluate the importance of within-ethnic-group variation affecting the person's orientation. 3. Consider the person's social class membership as a mediating factor. 4. Select ethnically compatible solutions to personal problems.
Mezzo: The FAMILY, CLIENT GROUP, and CARE-PROVIDER TEAM
1. Assess the ethnically based dynamics of the family, client group, and care-provider team. 2. Assess the responsiveness of the group or team whose members may themselves reflect different ethnic orientations. 3. Evaluate the importance of such within-ethnic-group variation. 4. Consider class membership as a mediating factor. 5. Select ethnically compatible solutions at the level of family, group, or care-provider team.
Macro: The COMMUNITY, LOCAL AND NONLOCAL
1. Assess family boundaries with the larger community in intervention and planning. 2. Facilitate community responsiveness to ethnic cultural needs. 3. Be aware of local/state/national policies affecting the integration of the ethnic group.

Source: Fandetti, Donald V. and Goldmeier, John (1988). Social Workers As Culture Mediators in Health Care Settings. *Health and Social Work,* 13(3) (Summer):171-179.

About one-half of American Indian, Eskimo, and Aleut elderly live in rural areas (Damon-Rodriguez, Wallace, and Kington, 1994:57), yet formal home health care services often are lacking in rural areas (Kenney, 1993), meaning appropriate care may be unobtainable to ethnic elderly.

One consideration to take into account regarding ethnicity is that poverty rates are higher among all ethnic minority groups of elderly Americans than among white Americans, and many elderly members of ethnic minority groups have no "medigap" insurance to cover the coinsurance and deductibles of Medicare. Thus, formal home health services may be rejected in favor of informal family-provided caregiving, partly because formal services are not economically accessible.

A second consideration in deciding between home care and nursing home care is that most geographical areas of the United States lack "ethnic nursing homes." Thus, people who have never been socially intimate with "white society" are not likely to be comfortable in a nursing home where most everyone else is white, and where the type of food, language, and decor is *culturally dissonant* to the ethnic patient, that is, not culturally acceptable.

Apart from cultural congruity, some evidence suggests that African-American elderly, for example, have poorer health status than white elderly and that both classism and racism in the health care system play a role in this (Wallace, 1990).

A third consideration in deciding whether to choose home care or a nursing home is ethnic difference in perspective of the optimal way to spend one's later years: European-American elderly people tend to see this as being able to function normally; Chinese- and African-American elders usually see it as internal contentment and satisfaction, while Spanish Americans usually see optimal old age is being able to enjoy life, to be a active, and to be with family (Wallace, 1996).

Aranda (1996) enumerates the main "ethnocultural factors" that need social work assessment in the process of acquiring the needed information to develop an appropriate care plan (see Table 5.6).

TABLE 5.6. Ethnocultural Factors in Health Care Assessments

A. Language
B. Norms regarding hierarchical relationships
C. Cultural presentation of symptoms
D. Cultural views on mental illness
E. Appraisals of cognitive decline and "loss of faculties"
F. Reactivity to or tolerance of cognitive decline and personality changes
G. Coping styles and behaviors
H. Informal social networks
 I. Caregiving norms
J. Biomedical history
K. Death and dying

Source: Aranda, Maria P. (1996). *Implications of Diversity for Practice.* Presented on June 18, 1996, at the California Geriatric Education Center, Cultural Diversity in Aging, Faculty Development Program, UCLA.

All cultures have traditions concerning family responsibility for the care of dependent family members, especially elderly parents (Mindel and Wright, 1982). It is important for the social worker, during the home care assessment, to explore client and family attitudes and feelings concerning such family responsibility.

The literature indicates consistently that African-American families may underuse services that could enhance the quality of their care (Morrow-Howell et al., 1996). African-American clients and their families are significantly more likely to prefer home care over nursing home care than are white clients and their families. The reasons for this are not yet entirely clear (138). In addition, African-American clients use significantly less formal home health care services and significantly more informal home health care services than white clients after hospital discharge, yet they rate the quality and quantity of their care lower than whites (Chadiha et al., 1995). The practice implication of this finding is that discharge-planning social workers need to explore the realistic ability of the informal care network to adequately provide the needed services, not just whether such a network exists (238).

Another study examined caregiver practices of German, Irish, English, and African-American ethnic groups. One of the main differences found was that among African Americans, the amount of time the family caregiver devotes to caregiving is not related to the closeness of the relationship, while among the Irish, especially, hours of caregiving was inversely related to the distance in the relationship between caregiver and patient. This difference was attributed to the African-American tendency to include more distant relatives and even nonrelatives with whom they are emotionally bonded as "family," while the Irish have a tradition of "duty" to care for close relatives (White-Means and Thornton, 1990a). Furthermore, African-American family caregivers provided significantly more daily hours of caregiving than either German, Irish, or English family caregivers (White-Means and Thornton, 1990b).

Variation in reluctance to use nursing home care also was found among Japanese Americans, whose future intention to enter a nursing home rather than home care was significantly greater among women than men, among those with little or no social support system, and among those who were born in the United States and more acculturated to American culture (McCormick et al., 1996). Whereas only 12 percent would plan to enter a nursing home following a hip fracture, 53 percent would enter a nursing home if the disability involved dementia (McCormick et al., 1996:769). The authors noted that this high percentage of respondents intending to use nursing home care under certain circumstances may reflect the fact that King County, Washington, where the study was conducted, happens to have "an ethnically appropriate nursing home which is strongly supported by, and familiar to, this close-knit community" (McCormick et al., 1996:769).

In working with Asian Pacific Islander elderly, it is essential for social workers to be sensitive to the fact that this category encompasses at least twenty-six ethnic subgroups, which vary widely from one another in culture and socioeconomic status (Tanjasiri, Wallace, and Shibata, 1995).

Applewhite (1995:248) points out that Mexican Americans are more likely to accept needed health services if the formal caregivers are aware and respectful of the culture of the patient and family, with regard to folk healing beliefs and practices and to the values of *confianza* (confidence), *respeto* (trust), and *personalism* (holistic mutual sharing) on an interpersonal level:

> [Mexican Americans] may avoid needed health care (such as formal home health care or nursing home care) because existing health care systems, with their emphasis on efficiency and impersonality, conflict with their cultural values, particularly *personalism*. (252)

INTERDISCIPLINARY TEAMWORK

In most formal home health care situations, the "team" consists of a supervising physician, professional nurse, nursing assistant, and family caregiver(s). Frequently, interaction among them is limited to intermittent contact between the nurse and physician, between the nurse and nurse aide, between the nurse and patient and family caregiver, and between the nurse aide and patient and family caregiver. However, rarely is there any interaction between the physician and nurse aide, and because the medical model dominates formal home health care, the relationships among staff tend to be hierarchial—with physician "in charge," nurse reporting to physician, nurse aide reporting to the nurse, and patient and family caregiver interacting separately with each of them.

What was just described is not an "interdisciplinary team," but a multidisciplinary team, at best, of the matrix model type (Mailick and Jordon, 1977). Interdisciplinary teamwork is not a hallmark of home health service in the United States. However, it is common practice in home health programs in many other nations that have more progressive health care systems and is highly recommended by geriatric specialists (Kane et al., 1997).

An experimental study (Zimmer, Groth-Juncker, and McCusker, 1985) of a home health care team, consisting of a physician, nurse practitioner, and social worker, to determine whether home health care patients served by the team would have a significantly different outcome than patients in a control group reported the following: (1) the experimental group patients spent significantly fewer days in either hospitals or nursing homes, (2) both they and their caregivers expressed significantly greater satisfaction with the care received than did the control group, and (3) the patients were significantly more likely to die at home, when that was their wish. However, there was not a significant difference in costs or in health status outcomes.

There is wide variation across HHC agencies in their utilization of social workers. Medicare requires that a physician authorize social worker services to an HHC patient on the basis that the need be related to the patient's acute medical condition. However, because Medicare will only reimburse for psychiatric nurse services when a psychiatrist is involved, it could be easier to gain authorization for a qualified clinical social worker than a psychiatric nurse when psychotherapeutic service is indicated. Unfortunately, however, "turf conflict" between the attending nurse and social workers can lead to underuse of social workers in home health care because both registered nurses and master's-level social workers have been professionally socialized to see psychosocial assessment and treatment as their own domain (Fessler and Adams, 1985).

Despite the underuse of social workers in HHC and the barriers to effective teamwork, the NASW upholds the principle of the interdisciplinary team and describes its positive potential in Standard 4 of social work in home health settings:

> **STANDARD 4:** The home health social worker shall integrate social work intervention with that of other members of the interdisciplinary team.
> *Interpretation*
> The complex problems experienced at home by special populations should be assessed and addressed from a variety of perspectives. A collaborative team approach has the potential for being more comprehensive, more efficient and more responsive to clients' needs. The home health social worker must integrate the psychosocial plan and interventions with the other services being offered and educate the entire team to the psychosocial needs of the client and client's family. (NASW, 1987:30)

ORGANIZATIONAL CONSIDERATIONS

There is an apparent association between organizational type and the extent to which professional social work services are used. Public HHC agencies, such as through Public Health Departments and voluntary nonprofit HHC organizations are more likely to employ full- or part-time social worker staff, while the for-profit HHC agencies more often employ social workers only "as needed," determined by the physician, sometimes with the recommendation of the attending nurse.

Although, in general, social workers are underutilized by home care organizations, in 1995, the median hourly rate of compensation to social workers by home health agencies was $16.25, and the median rate per visit was $42 (National Association for Home Care, 1996:9), indicating that the median social worker home visit lasted about two and one-half hours.

Home health agencies must be certified by Medicare to be reimbursed by Medicare for skilled health care services. In 1994, about 40 percent of home care agencies in the United States were not Medicare certified and presumably were limited to providing homemaker-type services or obtaining out-of-pocket reimbursement for skilled care (Cox, 1992:179).

CLIENT PROBLEMS
AND SOCIAL WORKER FUNCTIONS

Client Problems

The NASW lists the social work and psychosocial services in home health care as focusing on the following main categories of client problems:

- Patient and family adverse reactions or dysfunctional adjustment to illness and changes in functional status
- Vocational and educational problems
- Financial problems
- Caregiving problems, including caregiver stress
- Inadequate housing and living arrangements
- Barriers in access to medical care, including transportation
- Relationship problems, including social isolation
- Physical, sexual, and emotional abuse and neglect
- Substance abuse
- Other psychiatric illness, including depression and suicide
- Potential for institutionalization (NASW, 1995:6)

These may be conceptualized as falling under the headings of (1) barriers to admission to the service or facility; (2) problems of adjustment to the service or facility; (3) problems of adjustment to the diagnosis, prognosis, or treatment/care plan; (4) lack of information to make informed decisions; (5) lack of needed resources; and (6) barriers to discharge from the service or facility.

Client Health Problems

Table 5.7 indicates a wide variety of health problems found among home health agency patients. Table 5.8 lists the ten leading causes of death in the United States.

It may be noted that the major primary health problems of home health agency patients do not correspond very closely with the major age-adjusted causes of death per 100,000 population in the United States in 1993. This presumably reflects the discrepancy between

TABLE 5.7. Primary Diagnoses of Home Health Agency Patients, 1993

Primary Diagnosis	Percent
Cardiovascular disease	13.0
Musculoskeletal and connective tissue disease	8.5
Other circulatory system disease	7.1
Diabetes	6.8
Cerebral vascular diseases	6.5
Disease of the nervous system and sense organs	6.5
Malignant neoplasms	6.2
Respiratory system diseases	6.1
Fractures	4.1
Decubitus ulcers	1.3
All others	33.9
Total	100.0

Source: U.S. Government Printing Office (1995a). *Health, United States.* Washington, DC: Author, 197.

TABLE 5.8. Ten Major Causes of Death in the United States, 1993, Age Adjusted

Disease Category	Death Rate Per 100,000 Population
Heart disease	145.3
Cancer	132.6
Accidents	30.3
Strokes	26.4
COPD	21.4
Other infectious/parasitic diseases	15.9
Pneumonia	13.3
Diabetes	12.4
Suicide	11.3
Homicide and legal intervention	10.7

Source: U.S. Government Printing Office, 1995b.

what often is functionally disabling, such as arthritis and diabetes, and therefore requires supportive assistance to function and what is most likely to be terminal, such as cancer, but not necessarily have a prolonged period of disability. One recent nationwide study found that the "patient's functional status seems to play a stronger predictive role in determining post-[hospital] discharge than do [disease] severity measures" (Kane et al., 1996:247).

The relevance of the client's health problem to the social worker in HHC is the issue of how the health problem impacts mental, physical, and social functioning, particularly activities of daily living (ADLs), and conversely, how the client's mental, physical, and social functioning impacts the health problem. This is the reciprocal biopsychosocial interaction:

> For the chronically ill, frail elderly, homebound person, every aspect of life becomes affected and possibly changed as a result of the illness. Family relationships which may already have been strained become more so. The patient not infrequently is pauperized by the cost of medical care, raising issues of self-worth, pride, and dependency. Preexisting personality problems can become exacerbated and feelings of anger, self-pity and hopelessness are common. Further compounding the problem is the frequent inability of the patient to perform simple activities of daily living such as eating, bathing, and toileting. (Jacobs and Lurie, 1984:89-90)

Client Funding Problems

One of the many nonhealth problems of clients needing home health care services is the current lack of financial resources to pay for services. Currently, a patchwork pattern of sources of funding for home care includes Medicare (Title XVIII), Medicaid (Title XIX), Title XX of the Social Security Act (Social Services Block Grant), Title III of the Older Americans Act (Garner, 1995:1629), and the Veterans Administration and Civilian Health and Medical Programs of the Uniformed Services (CHAMPUS) (National Association for Home Care, 1996:5-6).

As with other areas of health services in the United States, home health care has considerable gaps in covered services:

- If one is elderly or disabled and eligible for Medicare, HHC may be available if a physician documents the need for *skilled care* (i.e., needing professional services, such as those of a registered nurse, physical therapist, or speech therapist).

• If you are poor and eligible for Medicaid insurance in your state, you may be eligible for home care for either skilled care or homemaker/chore-type services, especially if you otherwise are likely to need nursing home care.
• However, if you do not qualify for skilled care and are not poor enough to qualify for Medicaid assistance, but are age sixty-five or older, your AAA (Area Agency on Aging) may have funds to help with personal care services or homemaking services.
• Depending on your state's plan for use of Social Services Block Grant Funds (formerly Title XX), you may qualify for some assistance to help pay for home care.

In any case, the chances are that the client will pay, out of pocket, a significant share of the costs of his or her home care. Among clients who received any paid home care services in 1992, the average cost was $3,100, of which one-third was out of pocket (Braus, 1994:45).

Family Caregiver Burden

Although several million Americans receive formal home care services, Karen Pace, Director of Research for the Washington, DC-based National Association for Home Care, reports that estimates indicate that at least two-thirds of all home care assistance is provided free of charge by family or friends (Braus, 1994:40). The same association reported, in 1993, that an estimated nine to eleven million elderly Americans need assistance to remain at home (Braus, 1994:41). Most functionally impaired elderly people rely exclusively on family and other informal sources (Wilcox and Taber, 1991).

Spouses, mostly wives, are the largest group of caregivers of elderly people, and adult daughters, the next largest group (Brody, 1981; Horowitz, 1984). However, single women devote more time assisting elderly parents than do other family members. Because society tends to see them as "the nurturers," women continue to carry the major load of elder caregiving, whether or not they work outside the home. Most family caregivers are, themselves, middle-aged or elderly; about one-third are middle-aged, and another 25 percent are age sixty-five or older (Braus, 1994:41).

Although home care tends to be presented as a way to reduce government expenditures for hospital and nursing home care, this public cost savings is often obtained on the backs of family members, often women. The cost to these volunteer caregivers can include time, loss of income and retirement funds, neglect of their own health, lack of recreation and social life, and postponed careers.

A survey reported in 1988 (Linsk, Keigher, and Osterbusch, 1988) found that thirty-five states, in addition to the District of Columbia and Puerto Rico, provide some form of financial payment to family caregivers for providing home care to clients when the client is a high risk for institutionalization, in spite of the fact that both Medicare and Medicaid regulations prohibit the payment of family members for personal care services (206). This funding mechanism most often is state Supplemental Security Income payments, and the amount varies widely across jurisdictions. However, only thirteen of the thirty-five jurisdictions indicated that they sometimes allow payments to family caregivers of elderly clients. More often, the client is a mentally or physically disabled nonaged person. Besides state SSI funds, other funding sources sometimes used for caregivers of elderly clients include Title XX Social Services Block Grants, Title III Older Americans Act, Medicaid provisions other than personal care, or state general funds. The Medicaid Home and Community-Based Care waivers appear to be an increasingly important source of coverage (209).

Barnes, Given, and Given (1992) compared four groups of family caregivers—spouses with children, spouses without children, adult children with siblings, adult children without siblings—and found that spouses were most apt to suffer damage to their own health, while adult child caregivers were most apt to experience feelings of abandonment, especially if they had siblings. The findings have implications for social work in terms of the importance of an early needs assessment in home care situations to assist the family with caregiving plans (286-287).

The issue of whether home care is less expensive than nursing home care apparently is complicated, with the answer depending on a number of variables. However, one study found that when formal home care services were provided, there was a tendency for informal caregivers to reduce their own free services and to substitute formal ones. Although this raises the immediate cost of home care, it may enable family caregivers to keep the patient at home longer, thus reducing long-term costs (Ettner, 1994).

Social Worker Functions and Interventions

According to Jacobs and Lurie (1984):

> The social workers become an indispensable part of the home care team. They are able to provide *counseling, assist* the patient *with concrete* financial, housing, and medical equipment *problems, advocate* for the patient with welfare, the health care system, Medicaid, *support* the patient in *compliance* with the treatment regimes, help the patient understand and *deal with* strained *family relationships and* help the patient be reconciled to *chronic illness*. Indeed, in the absence of good social work care, home care services can be an exercise in the application of medical technology, while the patient remains miserable, kept alive physically but in turmoil and suffering emotionally.
>
> Social work in home care, by providing services in the home, returns to the origins of the profession, to that subtle, artful blending of support, counseling and advocacy which social workers do best. (emphasis added) (90)

Garner adds that other commonly needed social worker roles and functions include (1) helping the clients and/or families cope with their losses, including anticipated ones; (2) promoting medical compliance; (3) psychosocial counseling as needed; (4) advocating on behalf of the clients or families; and (5) discharge planning when clients no longer need the HHA services or when they need another level of service, such as a nursing home, hospital, or rehabilitation center (1995:1632).

Silverstone and Burack-Weiss (1983) argue, as a rationale for social work in home care, that all human beings need someone in their life with whom they are emotionally bonded and on whom they can count to provide, or arrange for, their needs as they arise, termed "the auxiliary function" (11). This is a fundamental function that the social worker can provide when needed, alone or with other HHC team members and family of the client. This is an affectively and instrumentally *supportive* function, including both a supportive relationship and supportive roles, such as interpreting, mediating, advocating, and monitoring person-in-environment transactions (11) in collaboration with the client and family (22). The mobilization of helping networks, when needed, is a major function of the HHC social worker (23).

The NASW has noted the following about the social work function and role in home care:

> The social worker assists patients and their families to adapt and plan in the home environment. Relief of stress, crisis intervention, assistance with financial problems, advocacy with community agencies, information and referral, assistance with planning, emotional support, appropriate counseling, and interpretation of and education about family and patient's needs to other health care staff and services providers, are the components of the social work role in helping patients adjust to their situations and in helping families sustain the patient at home rather than resort to premature or unnecessary institutionalization. (NASW, 1987:28)

In addition, the NASW Standard 6 for social work in home health settings (1987:30) states that the functions of the social worker in home health settings shall include specific services listed in Standard 4 of the "core standards" for social work in health care settings (see Chapter 1 of this text).

Elsewhere, NASW lists the functions and services provided by social workers in home health care as follows:

- Assess social, economic, environmental, and emotional factors that interfere with patient and family adjustment to illness and treatment.
- Explain social work services and contract goals with patient and family and develop a treatment plan.
- Provide counseling for long-range planning and decision making.
- Provide counseling, education, and support to the patient and his or her family related to the identified medical condition.

- Identify and obtain needed community resources on behalf of the patient.
- Advocate for services for patients at risk due to mental or physical limitations.
- Provide short-term therapy.
- Provide consultation, liaison, and interdisciplinary collaboration.
- Provide discharge planning. (NASW, 1995:5)

Case Management in Home Care

Ideally, social workers ought to play a major role as case managers in home health care. Who knows better than social workers how to gather important information from relevant sources to assess the needs and resources of a client and then to engage the variety of appropriate community resources to help meet those needs? Who can better work cooperatively with clients, professionals, and paraprofessionals from various disciplines to coordinate the timely provision of those resources and to provide ongoing monitoring to ensure their continued appropriateness, making adjustments as needed.

The broker role. A primary role of the HHC social worker ought to be that of a broker, a part of being a case manager, to link the client and/or family with needed community resources, such as a support group, home-delivered meals, chore services, telephone reassurance, volunteer home visiting, adult day care, medical aids and appliances, home modification/environmental adaptation services, or respite care (Garner, 1995:1632).

Ensuring the timely delivery of home care services. The social worker who does discharge planning in a hospital or nursing home also impacts on HHC services, insofar as he or she often makes the referral to the HHC agency and has arranged for particular services to be delivered by a particular time. However, one follow-up study to monitor the delivery of timely and appropriate HHC services found that in 40 percent of cases, one or more services was not delivered as planned; yet most hospitals do not follow up with patients following discharge (Proctor, Morrow-Howell, and Kaplan, 1996).

Still, NASW's Standard 5 for social work in home health settings states the following:

STANDARD 5: The home health social worker shall work to achieve an appropriate continuum of care, assuring the clients of ongoing services to meet their needs.

Interpretation

The home health social worker must consider all social work services as part of a continuum of care including the family, referring agencies and institutions and other community social workers. When possible, he/she must work closely with initial referral sources to insure the patient an appropriate discharge plan and safe transition into the home. Likewise, prior to the discharge of the patient from home care, when indicated, the social worker must establish the necessary linkages to community resources, or other facilities to assure that needs are met. (NASW, 1987:30)

Needs assessment in home care. Of course, the first step in case management is needs assessment, and the first issue in needs assessment is determining the appropriateness and feasibility of home care. Some of the considerations to explore with the patient and family that are relevant to deciding whether to opt for home care include the following:

1. Could the patient's condition be properly managed in the home?
2. Are there family members willing and able to provide the needed informal care (physically, emotionally, time-wise, in terms of other work and family obligations)?
3. If the patient and/or family prefers home care over nursing home care, what are the reasons?
4. Is the patient eligible for any third-party payment of any needed skilled care?
5. If not, is the patient or family willing and able to pay, out of pocket, for the needed skilled care?
6. Would the patient and/or potential family caregiver prefer the patient enter a nursing home facility, if one were available that was culturally appropriate and/or provided high-quality care in the community?
7. Does the potential family caregiver really *want* to assume responsibility for the informal care of the patient, or does he or she simply feel that it is "expected" of him or her?

8. Does the patient and/or family have any strong preferences or prohibitions concerning the gender or ethnicity of the formal caregivers provided by the HHC agency?
9. Are there any cultural values, beliefs, customs, prohibitions, and so forth, of the patient or family that the HHC agency ought to know about, ones that might affect the acceptability of the formal services to the patient?
10. What is the patient's and family's interpretation of the meaning of the patient's health problem(s)? That is, what do they think contributed to it and what do they think needs to be done to best deal with it?
11. Are the types of care services that the family caregiver will have to provide compatible with the family's cultural traditions concerning intrafamily relationships (for example, a daughter bathing her father's genital area)?

The home care assessment serves a dual function with elderly clients. It provides essential information for understanding their problems, needs, resources, coping mechanisms, and strengths. It also acts as a tool that enables clients to experience a "life review," which can help to achieve "ego integrity" (Erikson, 1950), or a sense of wholeness and fulfillment, after telling their life stories to an interested and empathetic listener (Kerson and Michelsen, 1995).

Social work in home health care should begin with a thorough psychosocial assessment, except in crisis-intervention situations such as elder abuse (Garner, 1995:1632; Silverstone and Burack-Weiss, 1983). The social worker assessment of the home care situation should, as always in contemporary social work, identify and understand both needs and strengths of the client system (Cox, 1992:180).

Depending on which other team members participate, the social worker's assessment may include, not only the customary psychosocial areas of the client's history and current status, relationships, and significant life events, but also ADL functioning, assessment of need for modification of the home environment, for support services, for income supports, for tools and equipment, and for interpersonal supports.

Activities of daily living status (eating, dressing, bathing, walking, transferring, toileting, going outside) and instrumental activities of daily living (doing housework, cooking, shopping, driving, paying bills, banking, etc.) are the primary determinants of the need for environmental modifications, support services, income supports, tools and equipment, and interpersonal supports. In fact, ADL status is one of the main determinants of the need for home care service (Fredman, Droge, and Rabin, 1992).

Assessment of mental status is also often desirable, since it is not always obvious how well oriented, depressed, or forgetful a person is, and these are common problems in older adults, especially among those who have been hospitalized and traumatized by medical procedures and by being in a strange and often frightening environment such as a hospital or nursing home. Depression alone is common among home care clients, who often experience a devastating sense of loss and of dependency. The outcome of an assessment of mental health status should be an important determinant of the service plan (see Table 5.9).

TABLE 5.9. Psychosocial Assessment of the Home Health Client

Traditional Psychosocial History Areas
Childhood family history and significant experiences
Marital family history
Educational history
Occupational and retirement history, income and insurance
Current household and housing situation
Transportation resources
Health history and development of current health status
Current support system, formal and informal
Religious status and preference
Political status and preference
Recreation, talents, special interests, pastimes
Reflections
HHC Supplementary Assessment Areas
ADL functioning
Mental status exam
Customary coping style
Specification of what family caregivers can/will do
Tools and equipment needs assessment
Support services needs assessment
Home environment modification needs assessment
Income support needs assessment
Interpersonal support needs assessment

A variety of assessment instruments are available to examine ADL functioning, such as OARS, or Older Americans Research and Service Center Instrument (Duke University Center for the Study of Aging and Human Development, 1978).

Assessment skills include empathetic communication, verbal following, synthesization of information, and ongoing feedback/evaluation (Aranda, 1996).

Client Outreach and Advocacy in Home Care

Many people, especially elderly people, who develop functional impairments do not know the available community resources, or are reluctant to ask for help (Blazer, 1988). Thus, the HHC social worker should ensure that the community has outreach services through, for example, the mass media, physicians, housing managers, postal carriers, hospital emergency rooms, and elders themselves, to provide information and referral for needed services (Silverstone and Burack-Weiss, 1983:27).

Advocacy is often related to outreach and is an important role for social workers in home care. Given the fact that most home care is provided by family and friends without benefit of formal HHC services, it is likely that many of these informal HHC situations involve either caregivers or care receivers who need someone to both reach out to them and advocate for them. Family caregivers often overwork and become overtired and even damage their own health unless someone reaches out to them and offers to advocate for them, whether with the care recipient, with other family members, with HHC agencies, with the family physician, or with politicians. At the same time, care recipients sometimes accept services of family caregivers or of formal home care agencies when they would prefer a different arrangement, but hesitate to complain when they are so dependent.

Advocacy is especially needed with vulnerable groups of patients, such as those with AIDS (Marder and Linsk, 1995). It has been a long, slow process in the United States to get nursing homes and home health care and hospice programs to accept and to treat AIDS patients properly, and the "battle" is not over yet. Advocacy may require education and information to correct misunderstandings, teaching new skills to deal competently with a new situation, pointing up the advantages of a previously rejected alternative, as well as using the force of law, when it is on your side.

The National Association of Social Workers includes as a specific service to be provided by social workers in any health care setting, "Client advocacy within and outside the organization, including attention to fiscal constraints" (NASW, 1987:6).

Counseling in Home Care

Kerson and Michelson (1995) describe the counseling work of a hospital-based Elder Care Center providing case management services that serves individuals and agencies throughout the entire county where it is located and whose services are reimbursed by Medicare. Their premise is that elderly people, regardless of their physical limitations, are still capable of introspection, of learning from past experience, and of psychological and social growth (160).

A primary goal of the Elder Care Center (Kerson and Michelson, 1995) is to help frail elderly people to remain in their own homes as long as it is safe for them to do so and to empower them to maintain the highest level of independence that their mental and physical status allows (160).

Some of the counseling activities provided by the Elder Care Center include the following:

1. Efforts to help family members understand the importance of the client's maintaining control over decisions about accepting needed services
2. Building a relationship of trust and mutual respect with "guarded" elders
3. Using pet therapy to "engage" certain clients
4. Helping the client to understand the family caregiver's need for relief through accepting supplementary services
5. Using life review and reminiscence therapy to facilitate "ego integrity" and reduce the dread of death
6. Engaging a resistant client in accepting a needed environmental modification to enhance quality of life, such as a ramp for a wheelchair-bound client

7. Using positive imagery and the relaxation response to reduce depression and anxiety, as well as the provision of "books on tape" and a tape player to help pass the time enjoyably
8. Helping the client to reinstate ties with some once-important sources of support, such as a former clergyperson
9. Working with family caregivers to reduce stress, through prioritizing and partializing problem sources and selecting alternative solutions, through expressing and examining emotions causing distress, and by linking caregivers with caregiver support groups.

The challenge of counseling in home care is to be able to work with both client and caregivers and to enable both to feel cared about, while supporting the primary client (Kerson and Michelson, 1995:183).

It is important to remember that people who are in need of home health care often are experiencing increased dependency and may not readily accept offers of various kinds of "help." The acceptance of dependency and assistance to compensate for one's dependency can be emotionally threatening (Cox, 1992).

Thus, it is essential for the social worker to be sensitive to this resistance to dependency and to provide counseling to support the patient and family with their decision-making process and in coming to terms with the need for supportive services (Simmons, 1994). A "cognitive therapy" approach might be useful here to help the client and family become aware of the meaning to them of dependency and acceptance of help, as well as to assist them in reexamining and reshaping those interpretations to become more realistic and generous to themselves.

Policy Activism

It is not enough that social workers advocate at the micro level; it is vital that social workers also voice their views about the current status of home care and the need to develop a model of home care that recognizes the significance of social needs as contributing factors to dependency. The first task of social workers must be to lobby for, make recommendations regarding, and participate in the design of a more humane policy, with appropriate program reforms, that promotes a client's right to live as autonomously as possible in the community (Cox, 1992:182).

NASW's Standard 2 asserts the following regarding home health care:

> **STANDARD 2:** Social workers in home health settings should support and advocate for appropriate home health care for people with chronic, acute, and/or terminal illnesses.
> *Interpretation*
> . . . Home health care social workers must be advocates for the maintenance of these individuals, families, agencies and the community resources and programs to support them. Advocacy must also be pursued on a state and federal level in support of legislation promoting home care. (NASW, 1987:29)

KNOWLEDGE REQUIREMENTS

Besides knowledge of social worker roles, functions, and service interventions, NASW has stated the following:

> **STANDARD 1:** Social workers in home health settings shall have knowledge of chronic, acute and terminal illnesses, physical disabilities and the resultant age-specific impact on individual and family systems.
> *Interpretation*
> Social workers in home health agencies must have knowledge of acute, chronic, and terminal illnesses as well as permanent and temporary disabling conditions. They must be familiar with the usual course of the illness or condition, therapeutic interventions, and adaptations which will be necessary by clients and their families. Social workers must also be familiar with the general concerns of special populations. They must be aware that these illnesses are often long-term and permanent, resulting in functional losses, social isolation and economic pressures which can impact on the individual's and family's ability to cope. (NASW, 1987:28-29)

Again, these areas may be classified under the need for specific knowledge of (1) the client population and client problem(s); (2) the organizational setting; (3) the community and its resources; (4) the needed research, evaluation, and documentation; and (5) appropriate intervention modalities.

Client Population

Home health care has a gender-specific, gerontological focus, consisting primarily of elderly unmarried women (Kaye and Davitt, 1995).

In 1994, about 1.9 million persons in the United States were under the care of a home health agency on a given day. Of these patients, about 73 percent were sixty-five years of age and over and about 67.5 percent were women. (U.S. Government Printing Office, 1995b:134).

Age and Sex

As age increases, especially among elderly women, home health care utilization increases. Among both men and women in 1993, the home care utilization rate was 3 per 1,000 among those forty-five through sixty-four, but 80 per 1,000 among men age eighty-five and older and 132 per 1,000 among women eighty-five and older (see Table 5.10).

The greater tendency of elderly women than elderly men to use home health agency services is largely attributed to the fact that old men are more likely than old women to have informal caregivers, that is, to be married.

TABLE 5.10. Home Health Care Agency Utilization Rate in the United States, 1993, by Age and Sex, Per 1,000

Age	Sex	
	Women	Men
45 through 64	3	3
85 and over	132	80

Source: U.S. Government Printing Office (1995a). *Health, United States.* Washington, DC: Author, 53.

In 1993, 25 percent of home health agency patients were under age sixty-five and the remaining 75 percent were age sixty-five or older (see Table 5.11). While the *rate* of home health agency services is highest among people age eighty-five and older, most HHA patients are under age eighty-five, presumably because the death rate has reduced the old-old age cohort.

Race and Marital Status

In 1994, in addition to the population of home health agency patients being primarily elderly and female, 63.3 percent of HHC agency patients were white, 15.9 percent were black, and the other 20.8 percent were of undetermined race (U.S. Government Printing Office, 1995b:134).

Also, 30.6 percent were married, 36.2 percent widowed, 16.7 percent never married, 4.7 divorced or separated, and the balance, 11.7 percent, were of unknown marital status (U.S. Government Printing Office, 1995b:134).

Since about 75 percent of the U.S. population was classified as white in 1995, and an even higher percentage of the sixty-five and over population are white, these data suggest that whites are underrepresented among home health agency patients. This may reflect a higher rate of functional impairment among elderly blacks and Hispanics and/or may suggest that nonwhites are more likely to use home care than nursing home care services (Morrow-Howell et al., 1996).

TABLE 5.11. Admission Age of Patients to Home Health Service, 1993

Age at Admission	Percent of Patients
under 65 years	25.0
65 years and older	75.0
65 through 74	24.2
75 through 84	32.0
85 and over	18.8
	75.0

Source: U.S. Government Printing Office (1995a). *Health, United States.* Washington, DC: Author, 197.

That the majority of home care clients are not married reflects the greater likelihood of needing formal services when one is unmarried. As Kane and colleagues (1996) recently reported, in a nationwide study of predictors of posthospital care destination, "Thus, the availability of informal care, at least as reflected in a person's not living alone, appears to play a substantial role in discharge decisions" (247).

One study comparing the characteristics of elderly home care clients who received formal home care services with those who relied solely on informal helpers found that formal home care recipients had far more fragile informal helping networks, which may help explain why they turned to formal HHC initially (Wilcox and Taber, 1991:258). In addition, the closer the biological relationship, and especially the closer they live to the elderly client, the more help provided by informal caregivers (259). Still, 32 percent of elderly persons in solely informal home care situations were receiving their assistance from non-family members (261). There was little or no evidence that formal HHC tended to reduce informal helping (264).

The Organizational Setting

As we have indicated elsewhere, social workers considering employment with a home health care setting need to know the organizational characteristics before accepting the position, such as whether it is a public or private, voluntary (nonprofit), or proprietary (for-profit) agency, what its history and current practice is in terms of use of social workers, degree requirements for social worker staff, and role expectations relative to other professional staff.

In addition, the prospective HHC social worker ought to explore what, if any, unusual limitations may be imposed on social work practice as a result of agency policy, secondary to its auspice or affiliation, for example, religious dogma, or secondary to its organizational priorities, for example, profit making.

The Community and Its Resources

As in all settings of social work practice, it is essential that the social worker be very familiar with the nature of the community and its resources, a phenomenon that is in constant flux and therefore requires ongoing updating of information.

Every community has a set of both formal and informal resources. The formal ones are the official resources, whereas the informal ones often are learned about through word of mouth. These may exist to serve the members of a particular religious, ethnic, or occupational group, they may be available in a crisis to supplement the formal resource system when it fails, or they may be ones that special individuals in the community sometimes give, under special circumstances, which are not widely known.

There is a rural-urban variation in the pattern of use of Medicare home health care services, including medical social work services (Kenney, 1993). Urban use rates are 9.1 percent higher than rural use rates. Population density is directly correlated with HHC use, and the number of nursing homes per Medicare enrollee is inversely correlated with HHC use rate. Rural areas have lower Medicare reimbursement ceilings, proportionately fewer visiting nurses associations, and lower availability of auxiliary services, such as medical social work, and physical, occupational, or speech therapy. Whereas 21.8 percent of urban Medicare-certified home health care agencies reported that medical social services were "not available," 62.7 percent of such agencies in rural areas reported the unavailability of medical social work services through their agency (Kenney, 1993:413). Kenney commented:

> . . . the consequences for rural residents of the more limited availability of auxiliary services such as physical therapy and medical social services need to be assessed. What happens when the rural elderly need these services? Do they enter nursing homes? Or is there an unmet need for these services? (1993:413)

Needed Research, Evaluation, and Documentation in Home Care

Knowledge of research is needed by social workers in home health care, as in all settings of social work practice. In particular, experimental design/clinical trials research is needed to test the efficacy of social work interventions. Our efficiency-oriented health care policymakers are not impressed with claims to effectiveness that are not supported by research (Ell, 1996).

In addition, monitoring the quality of home care is especially important because much of the care is being provided by nursing assistants with limited training, who often are without anyone to assist or oversee their actions or judgments. One process-oriented quality of home health care study found that 14.4 percent of reviewed cases of services provided by forty-seven different HHC agencies had quality-of-care deficiencies (Jette, Smith, and McDermott, 1996).

Kramer and colleagues (1990) propose a conceptual framework for assessing the quality of home health care that focuses mainly on two of three quality control measures, *process* and *outcome*, and to some extent the third, *structure*; they also think that HHC patients should be classified into homogeneous quality indicator groups (QUIGs).

The selection of outcome measures should reflect outcomes on which HHC can reasonably be expected to impact, and this varies with diagnostic category. For example, for patients recovering from a hip fracture, functional status (e.g., bathing, dressing, walking) is an appropriate outcome measure, whereas for a patient with heart failure or diabetes, level of knowledge, compliance, and ability to take medications are more appropriate outcome measures (Kramer et al., 1990:416).

On the other hand, for patients whose outcome is difficult to measure, such as the mentally impaired or terminally ill, it is more appropriate to examine the *process* of HHC service delivery, that is, the extent to which the services were actually provided, such as comparing the frequency of provided services with the standard for that service frequency, which many individual HHC agencies and associations of HHC agencies have developed (Kramer et al., 1990:417).

Structural standards for measuring outcome include such things as guidelines for organizational structure, qualifications of various types of staff, admission and discharge procedures, record keeping, and the provision of medications or equipment. These standards are useful indicators of organizational infrastructure, but are generally weak indicators of quality of delivered services (Kramer et al., 1990:418). Such structural standards have been developed by a variety of organizations, including the Joint Commission on the Accreditation of Healthcare Organizations (JCAHO), National League of Nursing (NLN), Texas Association for Home Health Agencies, and Colorado Association of Home Health Care Agencies (442-443).

Kramer and colleagues offer sixteen categories of HHC patient conditions most commonly reimbursed by Medicare (1990:421) and a table for each category that lists the suitable outcome and process indicators. Among the outcome indicators that could be relevant to social work interventions are client knowledge, compliance, family/caregiver strain, and client satisfaction.

However, according to Lawlor and Raube (1995), currently there is a "second stage" of health care outcomes research in progress, with a variety of disciplines involved, whose focus is on studying the cost-effectiveness of intervention outcomes to deal with health problems having a complex etiological mix of biopsychosocial factors as well as a complex mix of medical and psychosocial interventions. This approach appears directed toward producing specific protocols for specific health problems and has emerged in response to the discovery that medical interventions vary widely across geographical areas and providers. Furthermore, the psychosocial variables to be measured are not always observable in the individual, but instead in terms of family supports, culture, community, and environment (391).

A thirty-six-item, short-form (SF-36) instrument (Ware and Sherbourne, 1992) is available that serves to standardize and assess *eight dimensions of health status and functioning:* (1) physical functioning, (2) role limitations due to physical problems, (3) social functioning, (4) bodily pain, (5) mental health, (6) role limitations due to emotional problems, (7) vitality, and (8) perceptions of general health (Lawlor and Raube, 1995).

Because the causes of health problems are often a mix of biopsychosocial factors, the interventions and research often need to employ a biopsychosocial approach too (Lawlor and Raube, 1995). The first step in such interdisciplinary research is to *describe* what the various professionals and paraprofessionals actually do in community health care settings, and later to compare their efficacy in addressing particular situations. The trend is toward measuring such patient outcomes as quality of life, patient satisfaction, and social functioning, especially in home care and hospice care (395).

Lawlor and Raube (1995) note the intimidating complexity of the variables that need to be concomitantly examined to determine the outcome of home health care interventions. They present a framework for the design of such research with five sets of variables:

1. Client characteristics (health status, economic status, social support, sociocultural and home environment)
2. Organizational characteristics (structure, sponsorship, incentives for employees working in the home, organizational culture, and community environment)
3. Provider characteristics (specialty, education, age, gender, race/ethnicity, and practice tenure)
4. Intervention characteristics (cost, quality, complexity, instrumentation, and compliance)
5. Outcomes characteristics (functional status, satisfaction, quality of life, medical outcomes, caregiver burden, and utilization) (398)

The medical effectiveness movement poses a reasonable and traditional evaluation question: Which health care interventions work (Lawlor and Raube, 1995)? In spite of the complexity of such multivariate research, Lawlor and Raube advise the following:

> The individuals, disciplines, and professions who ask and answer this question will predominately set the standards by which care is delivered in the next 25 years. By integrating the expertise of social science, public health, and medicine, the effectiveness of health services that involve medical and nonmedical interventions and outcomes can be evaluated. (1995:401)

A "quick and dirty" approach to evaluation of HHC services for purposes of agency self-monitoring is proposed by Fashimpar (1991), who published such an instrument (Fashimpar, 1983), which both surveys consumer satisfaction and assesses progress on achievement of case and agency objectives.

The new HHC social worker needs to be sure to clarify the documentation requirements of the agency for purposes of reimbursement and Medicare-licensing review and to keep other team members informed.

VALUES AND ETHICS CONSIDERATIONS

Some unique issues are associated with home health care (Robbins, 1996:11-12), for example, the danger of theft of patient property by HCA employees:

> The home care environment offers greater autonomy for both patients and caregivers. This autonomy can be a double-edged sword. It is helpful sometimes not to have someone always looking over one's shoulder, but occasionally it is essential to gain access to guidance and support, something not easy to do in a patient's home. (Robbins, 1996:2)

Community-Based Ethics Committees

Robbins (1996) notes, for example, that home health care providers are often faced with the dilemma of patients needing services that are not reimbursable, yet the providers hesitate to complain to funding sources—such as Medicare, Medicaid, HMOs, or private insurance companies—for fear they will be seen as simply seeking to line their own pockets. He recommends the establishment of a community-based ethics committee consisting of representatives of local health care organizations, as well as a community leader and local clergy. Such a community ethics committee can help resolve particular case situations, propose agency and state policy for dealing with similar situations, and compile data from cases referred to them for use in lobbying (158).

Such a community-based ethics committee relieves the health care agency of having to deal with these kinds of issues and provides assurance to the patients, family, and the rest of the public that an impartial group of respected citizens is active in such decision making.

Advance Directives

The Patient Self-Determination Act (PSDA) of 1991 requires that all health care service organizations, such as hospitals, nursing homes, and home care agencies, at or near intake, obtain their patients' "advance directives" regarding their wishes for resuscitation, treatment, and life support measures under particular circumstances (Davitt and Kaye, 1996). Advance directives are written documents such as living wills and power of attorney for health care. Whereas the living will specifies one's own wishes, the power of attorney for health care allocates responsibility to a particular other person for making such decisions, should the need arise and one is incapacitated.

Depending on the legal requirements of the state and the policy of the organization, the social worker may be involved in interpreting the meaning of advance directives to clients and answering their questions and in assessing patient competence to complete such directives (Davitt and Kaye, 1996). Discussing these matters with clients and helping them to make such decisions and plans is an exercise in client self-determination and self-empowerment.

It is important that such directives be very specific as to the type of health condition for which one would expect to be treated and which conditions one would want to progress without intervention. When patients are mentally incapacitated, such as with Alzheimer's disease, the designated family member who is surrogate decision maker must make clear to the care facility and staff whether, for example, they do not want any curative treatment should the patient develop pneumonia, but would want treatment efforts should the patient fracture a limb or sustain a wound. Otherwise, nursing homes, for example, may simply assume that "no intervention" is desired under any circumstances, and later, the family members may experience distress that their loved one was allowed to suffer unnecessarily.

Advance directives need to be clear to all staff who will be caring for the patient and prominently located in the patient's room or on the cover of the care chart record. If a patient is transferred from one setting to another, it is important to be sure that the advance directives are transferred too (Robbins, 1996:7).

Analysis of Ethical Issues

Harry Moody (1982) has written about ethical dilemmas in home care and nursing homes; he uses an analysis framework from Reamer and Abramson (1982) that involves addressing the following issues in the process of resolving the dilemma:

1. Is the *source* of the dilemma the setting, the client health condition, or what? (What makes it a "dilemma"?)
2. Is the issue truly an *ethical dilemma or* simply a *practical problem?* (Is it that we don't know what we should do or that we know what to do but are not able to do it?)
3. How do the perspectives of the involved professions influence understanding of the issue? (*Are differences in professional values and ethics contributing* to the dilemma?)
4. What *level of action* is *needed?* (individual change, policy change, professional practice change)
5. How *do ethical theories clarify the dilemma?* (Does it shed light on the issue depending on whether you see it as one of rights, utility, personal virtue, or social justice. (emphasis added) (Moody, 1982:100)

SKILL REQUIREMENTS

A wide variety of skills is needed by the health field social worker. As stated earlier, any activity that the social worker performs in the course of his or her work may be "skilled" *if* it reflects social work knowledge, values, and ethics and is conscious, purposeful, disciplined, and responsible.

Simmons (1994) examined the future of social work in home care and described the following skill requirements for social workers:

1. Patient problems are multi-faceted and require services from a host of providers. Social work skill in complex care planning and service coordination is crucial.
2. The multiplicity of care providers addressing health and personal care are paid from a blend of public, private, and out of pocket resources. Social work knowledge of payment regulation is very useful in coordinating care. Experience with a full array of income levels is relevant as well.
3. Families provide vast amounts of supportive care. Friends and neighbors provide other informal care. Social work skill in

facilitating shared family decision-making and properly partialized caregiving is very useful. Family counseling skills are well used in this work.

4. Self-care is a critical element in managing chronic conditions to assure maintenance of maximum feasible health status. Social work health education and counseling skills are essential.

5. Mental competence, emotional and mental status are crucial factors in self-care. Social work skill in assessment, treatment, and other related skills are valuable with this population.

6. Health social work experience in facilitating interdisciplinary care planning for ethically complex situations, and facilitating patient and family involvement in decision making, is an important arena of professional expertise. (39-40)

COMMENTARY

Currently, we are in the midst of a period of rapid transition in health care, in which hospital social work, which has been the center of social work in health care, is undergoing downsizing as part of the "efficiency-oriented" health care cost-control process in the United States. At the same time, the center of health care is shifting to the home and community, where professional social work has not been officially recognized as essential to the health care system—*if* it is to achieve efficiency.

According to Simmons (1994), social workers may need to move into community settings, such as primary care physicians' offices, home health agencies, skilled nursing home facilities, residential settings, and adult day care facilities, in order to identify and reach out to people who need ongoing case management and assistance (41).

However, to achieve the objectivity that health care social workers need to be of maximum help to clients and to the overall objectives of the health care system, social workers may need to find some way to be independent of any particular sector of the continuum of health care organizations (Berkman, 1996).

When the social worker is employed by a hospital, nursing home, home care agency, or other organizational setting where social work is a "secondary function," some limits are imposed on what the social worker can do. For example, nursing homes have a vested interest in keeping their beds full, and so timely rehabilitation and discharge to home or to another less restrictive setting is not likely to be a high priority to management. Hospitals are eager to discharge patients ASAP so as not to exceed the DRG days and, if possible, to get the "profit" from releasing the patient before the DRG time limit. Consequently, rapid discharge planning becomes more attractive than quality discharge planning, which requires that the patient and family feel in control of the plan and are assured that arrangements are in place for continuity of care. Also, if for-profit home health care agencies are functioning in a highly competitive community, they may be tempted to retain patients in their own homes when either patient or family caregiver needs have emerged that indicate a transfer to a different care setting is required.

In any case, as Garner (1995) noted, "To date, social workers have played only a secondary role in home care" (1632). The main cause of this is that while Medicare mandates the "availability" of social work services to home health care agency patients, as needed, it does not mandate the participation of social workers in making client needs assessments. As a result, non-social workers determine whether social work services are needed. Medicaid programs vary across states, and there is no uniform requirement that social work services even be available in home care cases financed through Medicaid (Garner, 1995:1632).

Chapter 6

Social Work in Nursing Homes

HISTORICAL BACKGROUND

The Development of the American Nursing Home

Nursing homes in the United States today are a mix of proprietary (private for profit), voluntary (private nonprofit), and public (tax supported and nonprofit). The history of nursing homes in America varies with each of these three organizational types.

Public Long-Term Care Facilities

The earliest institutional form of care for the elderly, mentally or physically ill or handicapped, and other "dependent" persons in America was the variously termed county home, poorhouse, poor farm or almshouse. These were sometimes found in larger communities during the colonial era, but became the principle form of care of sick and otherwise dependent persons by the early 1800s—after industrialization, urbanization, and immigration incapacitated the earlier informal mechanisms of family and community care of the sick and needy. These were *public*, local tax-supported institutions (Boondas, 1991). In many cities and counties in the United States, these almshouses continued to exist until at least the 1960s (Dieckmann, 1993).

However, by the mid-1800s, there was widespread recognition of the unfit conditions in many such poorhouses, where "theory" and "practice" concerning the ability of the residents to take care of one another and to operate self-supporting "farms" proved to be discrepant. In response, during the latter half of the 1800s, many large specialized institutions sprang up, mostly *public,* state tax-supported facilities—such as for the mentally ill, epileptic, or mentally retarded. According to one psychiatrist who worked as an orderly in such a mental institution during the 1950s, these places served as much, if not more, to replace the "poorhouses" of the early 1800s in providing supportive care of the homeless, alcoholic, addicted, brain damaged, demented elderly, and other impaired people as to provide any specialized treatment for the population identified in the title of the institution (Vogel, 1991).

Voluntary Long-Term Care Facilities

In addition, by the mid-1800s, there began to emerge many benevolent care facilities for specific populations, sponsored by *voluntary* organizations—often with religious, civic, or occupational affiliations. Thus, "homes for the aged" sprang up—specific groups, such as for Germans, Jewish, Methodists, Lutherans, Baptists, Catholics, or Masonic homes, Elks homes, or teacher retirement homes. In general, the quality of care in such nonprofit facilities for the members of a particular subgroup was very good and set a standard for the care of the elderly as traditional nursing homes developed (Boondas, 1991).

Proprietary Long-Term Care Facilities

As early as the Colonial period, there also were some private for-profit boarding homes, which were the forerunners of today's proprietary nursing homes (Boondas, 1991). Such boarding facilities continue today, generally providing supportive, nonskilled care to mild to moderately impaired persons, while today's proprietary nursing homes are mostly classified as "skilled" care facilities.

As the United States entered the twentieth century, a variety of forces pressed for federal government assumption of responsibility to aid the elderly: the devaluation of the elderly with the transition from agriculture to industry and its emphasis on speed and efficiency, the reduction in extended families due to migration from rural to urban areas, and the transition to a wage economy with loss of social supports associated with close-knit rural community living. The Social Security Act was passed by Congress in 1935, providing for a variety of federal social insurance and public assistance programs, including a social insurance program of retirement pensions for the elderly, and the onset of "old age" was arbitrarily set at sixty-five years.

However, the Social Security Act stipulated that the Social Security pensions to the elderly could not be paid to persons residing in institutional care. The effect of this provision was an exodus of elderly people from institutional care to privately owned "boarding homes," some of which were operated by persons with at least some nursing training; such places came to be called "nursing homes" (Boondas, 1991).

In 1946, the Hill-Burton Act was passed by Congress. This act provided direct grants to public and other nonprofit organizations to construct nursing homes and other health care facilities.

In 1957, the Kerr Mills Act was enacted by Congress, offering federal matching funds to states to help pay for health care for the elderly and poor (Karger and Stoesz, 1994:282). These funds were often used to pay for nursing home care, then often provided in the nursing home operator's own home.

In 1958, the Small Business Administration was established and offered loans to nursing homes. These developments helped to meet the need for long-term care of the elderly, but also helped to promote the "medicalization" of the care of the aged (Boondas, 1991).

After Medicare and Medicaid were enacted in the mid-1960s, states transferred many of the residents of large state-supported institutions to nursing homes, in an effort to shift state costs to the federal government. However, another effect of the passage of federal legislation to provide public financial reimbursement for nursing home care was that many nursing homes were transformed from mostly small homelike settings into large, institutional, motellike facilities where rows of identical rooms, resembling the isolated cells of a beehive, housed "patients" to be processed in efficient assembly-line style. Thus, long-term care in the United States traditionally has been determined by reimbursement policy (Olson, 1994:31).

Olson (1994) also commented that

> The number of for-profit institutions in most other nations is negligible. As a result, no other country has developed the American equivalent of the nursing home; it is truly a unique institution. (33)

Funding Sources and Nursing Home Care

Medicare reimburses more generously than Medicaid because it pays only for skilled care. Consequently, many nursing homes prefer Medicare patients and avoid accepting those on Medicaid (Olson, 1994:29), producing a dual-track system of care (Boondas, 1991), one for the welfare dependent and one for the rest.

Even today, the best-quality nursing home care tends to be provided in retirement communities or "homes for the aged" that provide a range of care levels, including supportive living in houses and apartments as well as skilled nursing care units. These continue to be either the voluntary organizations that were started for members of a religious, professional, or civic organization or proprietary organizations for the affluent, both of which often require a substantial lump-sum payment upon entrance, in addition to monthly rates, with assurance of "lifelong care."

In 1994, the United States spent $949.4 billion for personal health care, of which 7.6 percent, or $72.2 billion, was for nursing home care (U.S. Government Printing Office, 1995a:244).

About 57.9 percent, or $41.85 billion, of the total $72.2 billion expended for nursing home care was paid for by the government: $34.27 billion, or 47.4 percent was paid through Medicaid for the indigent; $5.93 billion, or 8.2 percent, through Medicare for the relatively few who qualify for "skilled care"; and the other $1.645 billion, or 2.3 percent, through the Veterans Administration and state subsidies to hospitals (see Table 6.1) (U.S. Government Printing Office, 1995a:250).

Medicare expenditures for nursing home care are entirely for "skilled" care, which in 1994 was provided to 1 million, 26 thousand persons, age sixty-five or over, and to 42 thousand persons under age sixty-five with end-stage renal disease (U.S. Government Printing Office, 1995b:116).

TABLE 6.1. Nursing Home Care Expenditures, 1994

Payer	Dollars*		Percent	
Government	41.845		57.9	
Medicaid		34.270		47.4
Medicare		5.930		8.2
VA and other govern- ment programs		1.645		2.3
Out of pocket	26.846		37.2	
Private health insur- ance		2.202		3.0
Nonpatient revenues and industrial plant		1.360		1.9
Total	72.253		100.0	

Source: U.S. Government Printing Office (1995b). *Statistical Abstracts of the United States.* Washington, DC: Author, 115.

*In billions (e.g., 41 billion, 845 million)

In 1994, Medicaid paid for both skilled and intermediate nursing home care for 1 million, 639 thousand recipients, excluding the mentally retarded (U.S. Government Printing Office, 1995b:118). Medicare and Medicaid together helped pay for nursing home care for a total of 2 million, 707 thousand persons during 1994.

Thus we can see that the largest share (57.9 percent) of nursing home care is paid for through Medicaid—which requires that income and resources place an individual below the poverty line—and the next largest share (37.2 percent) is paid out of pocket. In fact, unless the individual is transferred directly from a hospital or within thirty days of being hospitalized and requires skilled care, that person is not eligible for Medicare coverage for nursing home care, and so must reduce his or her resources to at least the poverty level before becoming eligible for Medicaid.

Since the cost of nursing home care is between $100 and $500 a day (or $3,000 to $15,000 a month), it does not take very long for most elderly people to exhaust their life savings and enable them to become eligible for "welfare" assistance via Medicaid. For many elderly people, admission to a nursing home is viewed as close to death itself in terms of negative life events. If the elderly also must "go on welfare" to pay for nursing home care, the impact on self-respect and ego integrity can be tremendously eroding. Little wonder that many elderly nursing home patients have been found to be suffering from emotional depression.

If, as is widely contended, personal "empowerment" is essential for maximizing health status, nursing home care, as presently provided in the United States, is a major force defeating that objective. For-profit nursing homes have one overriding objective—to make as much profit as possible—and are therefore operated to meet the needs of administrators and stockholders rather than those of the residents or their families (Olson, 1994:32).

In 1991, there were about 14,744 nursing care facilities in the United States, excluding extended care facilities based in hospitals. Of this total, 10,522, or about 71.4 percent, were for-profit nursing homes; 3,497, or 24 percent, were private nonprofit organizations; while the remaining 725, or 5 percent, were public tax-supported facilities (U.S. Government Printing Office, 1995b:136).

Nursing homes are "big business" in America. If, in 1994, 71.4 percent of nursing homes outside of hospitals were for-profit enterprises and about $72 billion was expended in the country for nursing home care, presumably about $52 billion of the total went to the for-profit sector in revenues.

The nursing home industry is rapidly being consolidated into the hands of a few huge corporations (Karger and Stoesz, 1994:224-225). Furthermore, conglomerates unrelated to health care, such as Avon Products and Marriott Corporation have entered the market as well (Margolis, 1990:157, cited in Olson, 1994:32.)

In 1996, there were ninety-four U.S. corporations operating skilled nursing home chains. Four of these had combined revenues of 6 billion, 701 million dollars, as depicted in Table 6.2.

The Quality of Nursing Home Care

In general, nursing homes in the United States are sterile environments modeled after the interior appearance of a hospital, but without the quality of care provided in most hospitals. Instead, many nursing homes lack adequate rehabilitative services, mental health assessment

TABLE 6.2. Top Four Revenue-Producing Nursing Home Corporations, 1996

Company Name	1996 Revenues	Number of Employees
1. Beverly Enterprises	3,243,000,000	82,000
2. Manor Care Inc.	1,322,000,000	31,000
3. Sun Healthcare Group, Inc.	1,136,000,000	28,000
4. Continental Medical Systems, Inc.	1,000,000,000*	14,000
Total	6,701,000,000	155,000

Source: Wards Business Directory of U.S. Private and Public Companies (1997) (Volume 5). Detroit, MI: Gale Publishing Company, 115-116.

* Indicates estimated financial figure. Note that this fourth corporation is a subsidiary of Horizon/CMS Healthcare, which was eighth on the list of skilled nursing home corporations, with revenues the same year of another 639 million dollars.

and treatment services, meaningful social activities, or efforts to encourage decision making by the residents (Olson, 1994:34).

Most of the care is provided by laypersons with little or no training, such as certified nursing assistants (CNAs), and anecdotal reports from CNAs and family members indicate that state regulations concerning the ratio of CNA staff to patients per shift are not uncommonly violated, especially outside of the day shift during the week when there are fewer visitors.

Since the Omnibus Reconciliation Act (OMBRA) of 1987, nursing assistants in nursing homes must have at least seventy-five hours of training that addresses the nursing, psychosocial, physical, and environmental needs of residents, as well as medical needs, although many would agree that less than two weeks of training is not much preparation for the heavy responsibilities of the job (Kane and Caplan, 1990:277).

Use of chemical and physical restraints has been common in nursing homes. Although OMBRA, effective January 1989, was a major effort to reduce such abuses, mandating that such restraints can only be used in emergencies and only with the consent of the patient or family or by physician order, regulations have not resulted in major changes in institutional practices (Olson, 1994:35).

THEORETICAL PERSPECTIVES

An Alternative to Hospital Care or Home Care

Presumably, the basic rationale for having nursing homes at all is that some persons have health problems and accompanying functional impairments such that they do not require hospital care but are unable to be cared for at home. The reasons are because they are incapable of self-care, they do not have family or other volunteers who are willing and able to provide the needed care, and they do not have the financial resources to pay for round-the-clock formal home care services.

Because health problems and functional disabilities and loss of family supports tend to increase with advancing age, most nursing home residents are elderly. However, only an estimated 5 percent of all persons age sixty-five and over and 20 percent of the disabled elderly reside in nursing homes at any given point in time (Pepper Commission, 1990:92, cited in Olson, 1994:27).

Thus, most elderly people, with or without disability, live outside of nursing homes or other institutions, indicating that the decision whether to remain at home or to enter a nursing home is probably more a function of social and economic supports than of health status.

Cost Savings

Another rationale for nursing home care is that it is less costly than hospital care. Total expenditures for hospital care in 1994 reached $338.6 billion (U.S. Government Printing Office, 1995a:250), or 35.7 percent of the total $949.4 billion expended that year for personal health care, compared with 7.6 percent for nursing home care (244). Skilled nursing home care cost an average of $313 per day in 1994, compared with $1,756 per day in a hospital (U.S. Government Printing Office, 1994/1995).

The prospective payment system (PPS) enacted by Congress in 1983 is a system of predetermined payments by Medicare for hospital care, set according to diagnosis, known as DRGs or diagnosis-related groups. This system meant that hospitals could no longer keep patients as long as they saw fit and expect to be accordingly reimbursed, but instead had to discharge patients within a set number of days or not be reimbursed either by Medicare or the patient for the overstay days. Furthermore, discharge prior to the expiration deadline day brought the Medicare reimbursement for those "unused" days directly to the hospital as pure profit.

The Concept of Caring

Theoretically, nursing homes provide extensive supportive assistance to maximize the comfort and function (physical, emotional, and social) of their residents with chronic and/or terminal health conditions. This is caring at the third stage of health care. This type of caring means providing the patient with the tools and equipment, services, environmental supports, income supports, and supportive interpersonal interactions they require to maximize their comfort and function.

However, to some extent, nursing homes are expected to provide caring at the secondary level of health care as well. Since the prospective payment system (DRGs) began, acute-care patients are released from hospitals as soon as possible, and many are transferred as "subacute" cases to nursing homes to convalesce before returning home. These are not necessarily elderly people. In addition, many elderly people are transferred to nursing homes following such episodes as a stroke or hip fracture, not only because they need assistance to function, but also because they need physical therapy and/or speech therapy to be rehabilitated and able to return home. Such therapies or treatments are forms of "curing," whereas interventions to facilitate and encourage the accessibility and effectiveness of these therapies may be called "caring" or supportive interventions. Two-thirds of the people admitted to nursing homes stay less than three months (U.S. Government Printing Office, 1990).

The Medical Model

Although Medicare regulations require interdisciplinary teamwork to help implement a biopsychosocial perspective, neither the physical environment nor the program of most nursing homes is conducive to a "whole person" focus.

Presumably, the sterile atmosphere in many nursing homes reflects an attempt to resemble a place where people are not merely warehoused, but instead "treated," that is, to present a hospital-like atmosphere.

Patient rooms are generally furnished with the same type of beds, bedside tables, and chairs as found in hospitals. Floors are bare tile. Rooms usually are lined up along narrow halls, leading to the "nurses station," and so on. In short, the atmosphere in most nursing homes is not "homey," and it is not conducive to social interaction or personal empowerment.

In 1991, a nursing home resident, then age ninety-three, with a bachelor's degree in architecture, wrote an article (Mead, 1991) about his perception of the discrepancy between the type of atmosphere he had earlier enjoyed in a "home for the aged," which had since been closed, and that of the nursing home facility to which he was moved and in which he was now residing. He wrote:

> If we recognize that the primal nature of human beings is to seek fellowship, human understanding and inward comprehension, fostered by mutual inspiration and concern, then the nursing home becomes a very pernicious and inappropriate form of confinement (12) . . . while concentrating on the medical and habitational aspects of such facilities, the *in corpore* [physical] items mentioned earlier, we often overlook the *mens sana* [mental health] portion of the equation (14). . . . Maintenance of normal physical functioning can well be considered as primary, but without the assurance of being happy, competent and fully alive, to what degree can we appreciate good health? (15)

Caplan (1990) argues that most nursing home patients do not enter nursing homes to receive acute medical care, "yet the daily life of the nursing home is permeated by a model of staff-resident relationships that is firmly rooted in an ethic drawn from acute-care medical settings" (41).

HUMAN DIVERSITY RELEVANCE

In the better-quality nursing homes, homes for the aged, and so forth, due regard is given to the characteristics of the population being served. For example, Jewish elder care facilities have always tended to provide high-quality care, with well-trained professional staff, appropriate ethnic diet, and other types of consideration for ethnic-related preferences and traditions. Such consideration is more likely to be found in large cities where there are concentrations of specific ethnic groups, often with distinct languages, diets, and customs.

Unfortunately, where the population is predominately of white European background, and ethnic diversity is rare, members of such ethnically diverse groups are likely to encounter relative insensitivity to their preferences in the society in general, as well as in health care facilities, such as nursing homes.

Race and Ethnicity

Both hospitals and nursing homes were racially segregated in the United States until relatively recent years, and there is some evidence that nursing homes continue to be. This health care facility segregation was largely accomplished by the exclusion of black physicians from membership in the American Medical Association, resulting in their exclusion from practicing in hospitals that required such membership (Smith, 1990).

This continued for many years, even after the Hill-Burton Act of 1946 was passed, providing federal funds for hospital and nursing home construction, stipulating nondiscrimination but providing exception to this if "separate but equal" facilities were provided. Racial segregation in hospitals in both the South and North continued until the mid-1960s (Smith, 1990:564).

It was the NAACP (National Association for the Advancement of Colored People) and the NMA (National Medical Association), the professional organization of black physicians, that led the fight against racial discrimination in health care facilities (Smith, 1990:567).

It was not until 1963 that the U.S. Court of Appeals issued a majority opinion that hospitals were sufficiently involved with the state and federal governments to fall within the constitutional prohibition against racial discrimination. The surgeon general immediately issued new strict nondiscrimination regulations for those facilities applying for Hill-Burton funds (Smith, 1990:574).

These events were followed by passage of the Civil Rights Act of 1964, Title IV of which stated the following:

> No persons in the United States shall, on the grounds of race, color or national origin, be excluded from participation in or be denied the benefits of, or be subjected to discrimination under any program or activity receiving federal financial assistance. (U.S. Civil Rights Commission, 1963)

Finally, in 1965, Medicare and Medicaid were enacted, which raised the stakes further for hospital compliance with antidiscrimination laws. Noncompliance would have meant that patients could not use their Medicare or Medicaid coverage in the noncompliant hospitals, meaning both physicians and hospitals would have lost income (Smith, 1990:575).

However, the impact on nursing homes was not the same. These facilities were not eager to have poor patients covered by minimal Medicaid reimbursement, and they did not expect Medicare, with its restrictive eligibility, to amount to a very substantial part of their revenues (Smith, 1990:576). As it turned out, Medicaid expenditures to state governments spiraled much faster than expected, and since heightened efforts to ensure blacks had equal access to nursing home care would have meant even greater Medicaid expenditures, little was done to enforce nondiscrimination (577).

Although hospitals soon became subject to Medicare-compliance reviews, which further served to enforce racial integration in hospitals, nursing homes were not subject to such reviews. In 1989, the Health Care Financing Administration (HCFA) of the United States observed that

> Although in 1985 blacks constituted 31 percent of the Medicaid recipients and accounted for 21.8 percent of Medicaid expenditures nationally, they comprised [only] 8 percent of the recipients and accounted for [only] 8.9 percent of the expenditures for skilled nursing facilities. (HCFA, 1989:85)

In 1981, the Institute of Medicine noted that "most persons who have studied and written about black use of nursing homes believe that racial discrimination is a major explanatory factor" (Institute of Medicine, 1981:98).

While some people have argued that black families are more likely to prefer providing home care supportive assistance over nursing home care (Morrow-Howell et al., 1996), the Institute of Medicine noted that blacks are overrepresented in government psychiatric and chronic care facilities—which suggests that blacks will utilize services where they feel they will be accepted and respected (Smith, 1990:585-586).

Morrison (1995) reported similar findings among both blacks and Hispanics in New York City:

> Blacks represented 32 percent of residents in public facilities, 13 percent in proprietary facilities, and 11 percent in voluntary facilities. For Hispanics, the percentages were 8 percent, 1.5 percent, and 4.5 percent respectively. (Morrison, 1995:19)

Morrison (1995) questions whether America may continue to have a dual system of nursing homes, public ones for ethnic minorities and private ones for the white elderly. While these ethnic groups are represented proportional to their percentage of the total population, there is much evidence that their elderly populations have higher rates of disease and disability than their white counterparts (24).

Salive and colleagues (1993) reported a large longitudinal study to compare white and African-American elderly's use of nursing homes, and found that African-American elderly were admitted to nursing homes only about one-half as often as white elderly. The main risk factors for nursing home admission among whites were urban residence and mental health problems of a cognitive nature, whereas these were not found to be significant risk factors among African-American elderly. In fact, the study was not successful in identifying the determinants of the ethnic difference in nursing home admission rates.

Morrison (1995) proposed that the United States explore the feasibility of minority-owned and -operated nursing homes, home

care agencies, and other health care services for the respective
ethnic groups as an alternative to the current unsatisfactory situation.

While areas of the United States with sizable Jewish, Japanese,
Native American, Hispanic, and other ethnic populations sometimes have ethnic-specific residential care facilities for the elderly,
the difference in proposing separate facilities for African-American
elderly is that other groups have done it to more appropriately meet
the culture-specific needs of their elderly, who often speak a language other than English and have distinct foods and customs. With
black Americans, the rationale is more one of trying to ensure
quality care services in face of racial discrimination in the mainstream sector.

Social workers in health care need to recognize that, even when a
culture places great importance on family responsibility to care for
the elderly, as cultures change, the family members designated as
caregivers may experience considerable conflict between traditional expectations and present circumstances (Freed, 1990). For example, in Japan, one study closely explored the attitudes, feelings, and
behaviors of a set of families engaged in home care of an elderly
family member and found that (as in the United States) wives,
daughters, or daughters-in-law were the main caregivers, and in
most cases, they admitted that they filled the role reluctantly and
resented having to do so (Freed, 1990).

As in the United States, many Japanese women are now employed
outside the home and are better educated than before. Although
Japan has nursing homes, they are largely used for brief respite stays,
and nursing home placement of an aged family member is viewed as
a disgrace. Since hospitalization is not so regarded, many families
leave the elder in a hospital much longer than necessary to avoid the
conflict between home care and nursing home care (Freed, 1990).

Given that a family is now recognized as being a form of social
system, the assumption of responsibility for taking in and caregiving to an aged parent is often disruptive to that family system.

Another ethnic population in the United States that lacks access
to appropriate nursing home care is the Native American elderly
(Mercer, 1994). According to Mercer, 71 percent of Native Americans over age sixty have ADL functional impairments, yet there are

few nursing homes designed for them, and currently, most Indian elders who require nursing home care must leave the reservation and live apart from home and family. Unfortunately, most such facilities have no Indian staff who speak the resident's language, nor do they serve traditional foods or encourage traditional customs and needs, which can lead to social isolation and depression and an erosion of health status and quality of life (4).

In contrast, in the Navajo nursing home, at Chinle, Arizona, on the Navajo Reservation, described in the Mercer (1994) study, the elderly Navajo Indian residents are addressed by titles that they regard as endearing and respectful, are served Navajo foods, and are permitted to sleep on the floor in native fashion, if they prefer. All but two of the staff are Navajos. Although it is an intermediate care facility, residents appear comfortable and content. According to Mercer (1994), Native Americans have a particular need for more quality nursing homes that are culturally appropriate because many live on remote reservations where formal home health care services are not available, and where family members are often unable to care for them (Mercer, 1994). In this and another article, Mercer describes a variety of fascinating cultural characteristics of the Navajo elders she observed (Mercer, 1994, 1996).

The AIDS Stigma

Nursing home social workers also need to be sensitive to the problem of providing appropriate care for persons with AIDs, since the social worker often is responsible for admissions. Linsk and Marder (1992) found that hospital social workers rarely pursued nursing home placement for hospitalized AIDS patients upon discharge because previous efforts had met with universal failure. Yet, many such patients lack the financial resources or informal supports to enable home health care (106). This dilemma results in unusually long stays in hospitals, which is the most costly alternative in the health care system.

Linsk and Marder (1992) later found that new hospital social workers made extensive efforts to obtain nursing home placements for AIDS patients and were unsuccessful, while experienced social workers called upon lesser-known alternative resources in the community, such as specialized AIDS residences that could contract with HHC agencies. The authors report that the solutions obtained were usually less than were needed and lament the continued refusal of most nursing homes to accept AIDS patients. They also point out that nursing homes ought to be aware that the chances are that, unknowingly, they already have some patients with the HIV virus, and should therefore currently be enforcing the use of *universal precautions* by all their staff. Meanwhile, there is a need for specialized facilities for AIDS patients (Linsk and Marder, 1992:114).

In a letter to *Health and Social Work*, the President of the National Foundation for Long Term Care argued that, indeed, such specialized facilities for AIDS patients were needed, in the same way that not all facilities can provide all services, whether the service required is for AIDS, Alzheimer's disease, or ventilator-dependent children (Freeman, 1988).

This type of situation is one of many potential "ethical dilemmas" that nursing home social workers can encounter.

Sex and Sexuality

Since at least the late 1970s, the issue of sexual expression in nursing homes has been acknowledged (Kaas, 1978; Wasow and Loeb, 1979; Brown, 1989). A survey was recently conducted of social workers employed in twenty-nine randomly selected nursing homes in New York (Fairchild, Carrino, and Ramirez, 1996) concerning their perceptions of other staff attitudes toward resident sexuality. The social workers reported that all twenty-nine of the nursing homes studied allowed married couples to share rooms if both agreed; masturbation is thought to be the most common form of sexual expression among nursing home residents; and over one-half thought that the nursing home managers would not tolerate homosexual practice among residents. In addition, many respondents said they made no effort to ascertain the residents' sexual orientation. All but one of the nursing home social workers reported no formal policy or staff orientation regarding resident rights in the area of sexual expression, although about one-half indicated that the issue had come up in staff meetings. Fairchild, Carrino, and Ramirez (1996) offer some suggestions for development of in-service training directed toward clarifying specific resident rights in the area of sexual expression.

Although it is generally held that elderly nursing home residents need more privacy for sexual activities, a thought-provoking study of men with an average age of seventy, living in a Veterans Affairs Medical Center long-term care facility, found that when asked to rate the importance of "intimate" social, intellectual, emotional, or physical interactions, the men rated physical sexual intimacy as least important and social intimacy as most important. This was found among both married and unmarried men (Bullard-Poe, Powell, and Mulligan, 1994).

INTERDISCIPLINARY TEAMWORK

Nursing home regulations by both Medicare and the Joint Commission on the Accreditation of Healthcare Organizations (JCAHO) (1993) require that each patient has an individualized interdisciplinary plan of care based on a comprehensive assessment of patient health and psychosocial status. Social services are delineated as essential to the multidisciplinary care team and as having fundamental responsibility for the psychosocial assessment and for sharing in the meeting of patients' psychosocial needs.

All nursing homes that receive funds through Medicare or Medicaid are required to hold regular interdisciplinary team meetings within a few days of patient admission and periodically thereafter. The idea is that each key team member will conduct an assessment of patient status and needs in his or her own professional skill area and identify tentative objectives and associated interventions for that resident's care. This information is then shared among team members so that understanding and intervention are coordinated.

Nursing homes that expect to accept Medicare patients must be "Medicare certified" and undergo a survey by the Health Care Financing Administration (HCFA), the federal umbrella agency responsible for Medicare and Medicaid programs, at least once every ten months (Williams, 1997). However, the Joint Commission on the Accreditation of Healthcare Organizations is an independent, nonprofit organization and the oldest and largest standards-setting and accrediting body in health care, but nursing homes are not required to be accredited by JCAHO, and only about 10 percent of nursing homes have JCAHO accreditation (Williams, 1997).

Furthermore, JCAHO allows a variety of options in the provision of social services: a social worker who has completed the course work for an MSW from a CSWE-accredited school of social work, one who has the documented equivalent in education, training, and/or experience ("a qualified social worker"), or someone with a bachelor's degree, preferably with a social work sequence and additional on-the-job training ("a social services assistant") (JCAHO, 1993). A social services assistant must consult with a qualified social worker on a monthly basis.

If none of these options is selected, an alternative is to contract with an outside organization, such as a school of social work or community agency, that uses the direct services of a qualified social worker (JCAHO, 1993:53). Obviously, cost-conscious facilities under pressure to reduce "overhead" will tend to opt for the least-expensive alternative.

Finally, this writer has observed considerable variation across nursing homes in the quality of interdisciplinary (ID) teamwork. In some nursing homes, regular and frequent ID team meetings are held with a full spectrum of professional staff, who attend the meetings well-prepared to share with one another the results of their assessments of patients and their helping intervention plans. Sometimes a concerned family member and/or the patient is present and included with respect. At the other extreme are nursing homes whose ID teamwork practice is a "farce." These are characterized by irregular and infrequent team meetings, attended by few representatives of professional staff, who sometimes appear to regard the team meetings as a necessary, but annoying, government requirement and give little indication that they have developed, or intend to develop, thoughtful care plans.

ORGANIZATIONAL CONSIDERATIONS

Essentially, the extent to which interdisciplinary teamwork is a reality in nursing homes depends greatly on the extent to which the nursing home management values it as ideal and takes appropriate action to facilitate its working.

All health care settings are secondary or "host" settings for social work, and so the organizational mission is defined and dominated by other than social workers (Dane and Simon, 1991, cited in Kruzich and Powell, 1995).

Bureaucratization

Brannon (1992) wrote:

> From the viewpoint of the student of organizations, nursing homes are paradoxes. Although organizational size is usually positively associated with levels of bureaucratization, nursing homes are small organizations that exhibit decidedly bureaucratic structures. Families and residents experience bureaucracy in a variety of ways including: the routinized, sometimes "assembly line" nature of care routines; the highly regulated hierarchy of information exchange and authority within the staff; and the prominence of rules and procedures over negotiated relationships as guides for behavior. . . . Yet some nursing homes feel less bureaucratic than others. Examples of autonomy-enhancing organizational strategies have been cited (Kane and Caplan, 1990) and innovations within the industry are apparent. The challenge is for second-generation nursing home researchers to simultaneously look within and across facilities to identify patterns of organizational design, work design, and human resource strategies that enhance resident well-being. This will require cross disciplinary thinking, which results in studies of individual behavior framed in organizational context variables and studies of institutions attending to individual differences. (294)

Organizational Priorities and Objectives

Presumably, if the facility is managed by a business administrator, as for-profit facilities are likely to be, the organizational objectives and priorities will tend to diverge from those of a voluntary or public facility often managed by a health care professional, such as a registered nurse or MSW social worker. The organizational objectives of such professionals will tend to revolve around a greater commitment to a biopsychosocial and an interdisciplinary perspective directed toward a high quality of life and care of the residents.

Also, the less priority placed on financial profit, the more likely the facility is to employ well-trained professional staff who are dedicated to high-quality care and sensitivity to human diversity, who value the relationship between patient empowerment and patient health status, and who understand the need for nursing assistants to have a low enough patient care load that they can provide sensitive, individualized, quality caregiving that is rewarding for both patient and caregiver.

Authority Structure/Decision-Making Style and Sense of Empowerment

Some evidence suggests that the less a nursing home relies on a bureaucratic authority structure and the more the organization functions as a participatory democracy, the greater the sense of empowerment of the staff, including social workers. One nursing home study (Kruzich, 1995) compared perceived control of directors of nursing, directors of social services, activity directors, charge nurses, and nursing assistants over various areas of decision making. The study showed that the greater perceived influence of the nursing director, the less the perceived influence of the charge nurse; the greater the perceived influence of the charge nurse, the greater the perceived influence of the nursing assistants; and the greater the perceived control of the activity directors over resident care decisions, the greater the perceived influence of the social service directors over resident care decisions (210).

The three *structural variables* most associated with increased perceived influence of all staff combined were nonprofit organizational status, larger size facilities, and nonunionized facilities, while the *process variables* most associated with increased perceived influence were nursing assistant participation in shift report, more frequent staff meetings, and less rotation of nursing assistant staff among residents and units (Kruzich, 1995:213).

A study of nursing home social workers in Wisconsin found that of five broad areas of potential social worker influence in the nursing home, both the online social workers and directors of social work in the nursing homes studied agreed that the two areas of greatest social work influence were (1) care planning, including making changes in care plans and planning residents "care," and (2) resident transfer, specifically deciding if residents are transferred in or out of the facility (Kruzich and Powell, 1995:218).

The same study also found that social work directors in nursing homes perceived themselves as having more influence in publicly owned and nonprofit facilities than in for-profit facilities. Also, such facilities employed more full-time social workers (Kruzich and Powell, 1995:218).

Curiously, social workers employed in nursing homes with a resident council perceived themselves as having more influence than social workers in homes without a resident council, and the extent of perceived social worker influence was positively correlated with the degree of resident autonomy and resident satisfaction in the home (Kruzich and Powell, 1995:221).

Although it is not clear whether social worker influence is the cause or result of organizational flexibility and shared decision making, the findings indicate that the lone social worker in a for-profit facility is likely to be in a relatively powerless position (Kruzich and Powell, 1995). The significance of these study findings is that they provide some clues as to the impact of organizational variables on staff and resident satisfaction, which is believed to be correlated with level of perceived autonomy or influence, which is, in turn, associated with well-being and health status (Kruzich, 1995).

Use of Proprietary Nursing Homes As Settings of Social Work Student Practicums

A 1991 survey (Hancock, 1992) of MSW educational programs in universities explored their use of for-profit organizational settings for field placements and found that health care organizations were most commonly used, and the universities were fairly evenly split between whether they do or do not use such settings without restrictions or criteria. Over one-half, or 55.4 percent, reported using for-profit nursing homes for placements, and about 61.8 percent did so without restriction (334). Use of for-profit settings for social work student field placement was found to vary by geographical region, with the highest percent (57.1 percent) in the Southwest, followed by the

Southeast (43.7 percent), Mid-Atlantic (33.0 percent), West (28.6 percent), and Midwest (26.7 percent), with the lowest percentage in the Northeast (18.2 percent). Furthermore, the programs in the Southwest were least restrictive, while those in the Northeast were the most restrictive (335). In short, although most MSW programs in universities use for-profit settings for field placements, they vary considerably in their level of comfort with such placements (337).

Role Conflict and Staff Burnout

Another study (Barber and Iwai, 1996) examined the relative influence of (1) staff characteristics, (2) workload and caregiving involvement (emotional closeness with patients, number of patients cared for, and number of hours worked per week), (3) work environment characteristics (role ambiguity and role conflict), and (4) social support in predicting burnout among caregiving staff of Alzheimer's patients in nursing homes.

Role conflict, defined as two or more simultaneous expectations that are incompatible, such that performance of one makes it difficult to comply with the other, was found to account for most (56.5 percent) of the variance in likelihood of burnout. This implies that organizational strategies that minimize role conflict should effectively reduce burnout (Barber and Iwai, 1996:113). In addition, the findings underscore the developing conviction that both staff and patients/residents function better when they feel empowered and that a sense of powerlessness or helplessness is destructive to humans.

CLIENT PROBLEMS
AND SOCIAL WORKER FUNCTIONS

Client Problems

As previously suggested, it may be useful to conceptualize client problems in health care settings as the following:

1. Barriers to admission to the facility or service
2. Problems of adjustment to the facility or service
3. Problems of adjustment to the diagnosis, prognosis, or care plan
4. Lack of information to make informed decisions and take control
5. Lack of resources to meet needs
6. Barriers to discharge from the facility or service

In 1992, Vourlekis, Gelfand, and Greene provided a list of twenty-eight psychosocial needs of nursing home residents and families which

> ... was generated through a reiterated process of experiential and intuitive identification of issues on the part of a diverse group of nursing home experts, literature review in the psychosocial domain ... and critique and revision by the expert group. (114)

Thus, we present their list in Table 6.3 as a legitimate list of psychosocial needs of nursing home residents and their families that nursing home social workers should address.

Social Worker Functions

Vourlekis, Gelfand, and Greene (1992) also have provided the following list of twenty-three nursing home social worker functions that was developed in 1988 to 1989 by NASW's Nursing Home Clinical Indicator Work Group (114) (see Table 6.4).

The Vourlekis, Gelfand, and Greene (1992) study comparing the expectations of a sample of NASW member social workers and nursing home administrators for the social worker role in the nursing home setting found the following:

1. Nursing home administrators rated higher than social workers the importance of all but one of the listed "needs" of residents, family, and staff; they also rated higher than social workers the expected frequency of performance of the functions.
2. Some differences were seen in ranking of functions between the staff social workers and consultant social workers, with staff social workers focused more on direct services to residents and consultant social workers more involved in training and otherwise working with staff.
3. Administrators expected social workers to spend more time working with resident discharges than social workers reported doing.
4. Of twenty-eight psychosocial needs of nursing home residents, three of the five that both administrators and social workers rated most important were the same: (1) transitional support, (2) help with loss, and (3) relatedness and intimacy.

TABLE 6.3. Psychosocial Needs of Nursing Home Residents and Their Families

1. Emotional support in coping with the transition to the home.
2. Help with feelings of loss throughout the stay in the home.
3. Help with fears/anxieties . . . throughout the stay in the home.
4. Specific help in preparing for and coping with death.
5. Recognition by staff that "difficult behavior," including aggressiveness and withdrawal/apathy, may signify emotional distress, and need for interventions based on a specific understanding of that distress.
6. Help with financial planning and decision making prior to coming to the home, and assistance in locating and accessing financial resources at any point during the stay in the home.
7. Opportunity and assistance as needed with access to activities and events within the home which are diverse enough to match each resident's capabilities and interests.
8. Opportunities and needed assistance with access to outside activities and events.
9. Help with acquiring or replacing needed personal belongings or other practical transactions.
10. Choice concerning important daily routines.
11. Choice and control over decisions affecting care.
12. Recognition of need and opportunity to express religious, ethnic, cultural identity.
13. Recognition of status and wholeness of one's life history.
14. Ongoing relatedness and intimacy with family and loved ones.
15. Specific emotional support to family members/significant others in response to their needs or reactions.
16. Family collaboration in care planning and decision making.
17. Informal social opportunities with other residents.
18. Independence in functioning and opportunity to do for oneself whenever possible, whatever the level of functioning.
19. Structured social and group interaction opportunities both inside and outside the home.
20. Maintaining contact with friends/associates/community ties outside home.
21. Contributing to the life and functioning of the nursing home community.
22. In-depth orientation to the home, staff, policies, procedures.
23. Orientation to resident/family rights/obligations, and grievances process.
24. Family/resident input to survey/certification and accreditation process.
25. Opportunity for formal feedback to home personnel on level of satisfaction with aspects of home care.
26. Opportunity for structured dialogue between families, residents, and home personnel concerning care management.
27. Security that appropriate care will be in place at points of transition whether into, within, or out of the home.
28. Assurance that care/resources which are supposed to be provided, are.

Source: Vourlekis, Betsy S., Gelfand, Donald E., and Greene, Roberta R. (1992). Psychosocial Needs and Care in Nursing Homes: Comparison of Views of Social Workers and Home Administrators. *The Gerontologist,* 32(1):115. Copyright © The Gerontological Society of America. Reproduced by permission of the publisher.

TABLE 6.4. Nursing Home Social Worker Functions

1. Review appropriateness of admission applications and provide information and referral as needed.
2. Promote applicant's participation in the decision to enter the home.
3. Perform comprehensive social psychological assessment, including resident's preferences.
4. Help residents and their families cope with the immediate effects of the decision to move to the nursing home.
5. Orient residents and families to the facility.
6. Assist resident and family with financial planning.
7. Involve residents and families in care planning including their attendance at care conference if they desire.
8. Work with relevant staff to implement each resident's care plan, addressing especially issues that express and reinforce individuality and identity.
9. Enable social functioning using varied treatment interventions (group, individual, family).
10. Assist residents to adapt to living in an institutional environment.
11. Mediate issues that arise between and among residents, family, and staff.
12. Ameliorate emotional distress of resident and family.
13. Provide linkage with community resources by maintaining knowledge of other systems, making referrals/contacts, and identifying unmet needs.
14. Empower residents and enable maximum choice in matters affecting them.
15. Provide crisis intervention.
16. Help resident, family, and staff prepare for and cope with death.
17. Monitor the effect of governmental and facility rules and regulations and their interpretation on the everyday life of residents/families.
18. Affect facility policy/practice to promote choice in schedule and lifestyle.
19. Train, and consult with, other staff and volunteers regarding psychosocial needs of both individual residents and the resident group as a whole.
20. Advocate on a case level.
21. Advocate on a policy and program level.
22. Participate in policy decision making which affects resident care and family involvement.
23. Plan discharges with resident and family participation to assure continuity of care for transfers in and out and discharges from the nursing home.

Source: Vourlekis, Betsy S., Gelfand, Donald E., and Greene, Roberta A. (1992). Psychosocial Needs and Care in Nursing Homes: Comparison of Views of Social Workers and Home Administrators. *The Gerontologist,* 32(1):115. Copyright © The Gerontological Society of America. Reproduced by permission of the publisher.

Social Work Functions According to NASW Standards

According to Standard 4 of NASW Standards for Social Work Services in Long-Term Care Facilities:

> The functions of the social work program should include but not be limited to *direct services* to individuals, families, and significant others; *health education* for residents and families; *advocacy; discharge planning; community liaison* and services; participation in *policy and program planning; quality assurance; development of a therapeutic environment* in the facility; *and consultation* to other members of the long-term care team.

Interpretation

The social work program is directed toward providing services designed to identify and meet the social and emotional needs of each resident; to assist each resident and family to adjust to the effects of the illness or disability, treatment, and stay in the facility; and to assure adequate discharge planning and the appropriate use of community and social and health resources. (emphasis added) (1981:5)

Specific social work service functions include the following:

- Preadmission services, including psychosocial assessment and participation in interdisciplinary evaluation of the individual's need for institutional care and preparation of the incoming resident.
- Development of individual social services plans designed to meet the needs of the resident, the family, and significant others. The initial goals of the individual plan should be to promote adjustment and lessen the trauma of relocation to the new environment.
- Assistance to residents, potential residents, and families and significant others in finding and utilizing financial, legal, mental health, and other community resources.
- Provision of individual, family, and group services focused on the enhancement of psychosocial functioning and on social and

emotional problems, such as adjustment to illness or disability, institutional living, inter- or intra-institutional transfers, inter-personal relationships, reestablishing community living, and coping with separation, loss, dying, and death.
- Participation in the interdisciplinary care team comprehensive resident treatment planning and evaluation and coordination of patient care services.
- Advocacy of the rights of residents through the development and implementation of policies for the facility and self-governing councils, and assurance that guardianship, conservatorship, and case management services be made available to residents in need.
- Facilitation of the resident's integration into the community through discharge planning and followup services.
- Orientation and supervision of volunteers when appropriate.
- Participation in planning and policy development for the facility as a whole, including collaboration with other members of the staff in the identification of social, psychological, and cultural factors essential to the enhancement of the therapeutic and physical environment.
- Participation in orientation and in-services training of other facility personnel.
- Contribution to the development of community resources by participating with community groups to initiate, plan, and carry out programs concerned with the health and welfare needs of the target population.
- Supervision of fieldwork in affiliation with an accredited school of social work.
- Participation in research and demonstration projects that may be conducted either independently or collaboratively. (NASW, 1981:5-6)

To assist social workers and reviewers in monitoring and evaluating the adequacy of social services in the nursing home setting, the NASW has developed several "indicators," or benchmarks, for such measurement. Four of these indicators concern the *process* of social work services, and an additional two concern the *outcome* of such services.

According to NASW Clinical Indicators for Social Work and Psychosocial Services in Nursing Homes (1993:1-12) the four essential indicators of the quality of the *process* of social work services in nursing homes are the following:

1. Timely psychosocial assessment (Comprehensive resident evaluation occurs soon after admission to the home.)
2. Comprehensive psychosocial assessment (Resident's psychological and social circumstances are assessed adequately.)
3. Resident involvement in care planning (The resident is included in care planning and decision making.)
4. Family involvement in care planning (The wishes and thoughts of the resident's family are explored with sensitivity to cultural factors and lifestyle, and the family is aware of the care plan and decisions made by the care planning team.)

The two essential indicators of the quality of the *outcome* of social work services in nursing homes are as follows:

1. Resident satisfaction with choice (Residents are satisfied with the degree of choice available in everyday matters in the home.)
2. Problem resolution (Residents' psychosocial problems are ameliorated.)

The rationales for these six indicators of the quality of social work services in nursing homes follow, in order:

Rationale 1: Information and conclusions of a comprehensive social history and social and psychological assessment that includes racial, cultural, ethnic, and religious information and sexual orientation must be available on a timely basis to guide care planning and ongoing care provision.

Rationale 2: To adequately guide planning and decision making the psychosocial history and assessment addresses both needs and strengths (for example, assets and resources) in the resident and in his or her situation and spells out the implications of this information for care planning.

Rationale 3: The resident's plan covers matters that define the parameters of everyday life. It must reflect his or her preferences and choices, including cultural, ethnic, and religious background and sexual orientation. Residents or their surrogates must be aware of what is embodied in the care plan and must have the right to refuse aspects of care.

Rationale 4: Family input into care planning provides important information to guide decision making. Once a care plan is in place the family should be fully informed to enhance positive collaboration. The social worker facilitates communication between the family and the care team before and after the care-planning conference.

Rationale 5: Greater control over one's life is presumed to contribute to social and psychological well-being. Though social work is not solely responsible for positive or negative outcomes on this dimension, one function of social work is to identify preferences and individuality in the psychosocial assessment and to facilitate choices through working directly with residents and their families, educating and sensitizing staff, developing mechanisms for choice, and working at policy levels in the home.

Rationale 6: The intent of social work intervention is to help residents meet psychosocial needs and improve and solve problems related to nursing home life and care. Problem resolution is an indicator of whether the intervention has achieved its goal. (NASW, 1993:6-8)

KNOWLEDGE REQUIREMENTS

What Nursing Home Social Workers Say They Need to Know More About

Thanks to the Omnibus Budget Reconciliation Act of 1987 (PL 100-203), which placed renewed emphasis on the importance of psychosocial care in nursing homes, the position of social services in nursing homes has been strengthened (Greene et al., 1992). Medically related social and emotional needs of patients must now be identified, and a clear plan is required to assist each patient in adjusting to the social and emotional aspects of his or her illness, treatment, and stay in the facility (40). Every nursing home facility of 120 or more beds must provide the services of a social worker (40).

However, many nursing home social workers have no more than a bachelor's degree in social work or a "related field" (Quam and Whitford, 1992) and may be expected to assume responsibility for functions for which they are ill prepared. When 301 nursing home social workers were asked to rate a variety of subject areas by level of interest, relevance to job, and level of present competence, *they generally indicated a need to know more about behavior problems of the elderly, medical terminology and prescription information, mental health issues, cognitive changes in aging, and how to work with families* (Quam and Whitford, 1992:151).

However, even a survey (Greene et al., 1992) of 152 professional social worker members of NASW, who were employed by nursing homes, many as consultants, concerning the nursing home characteristics, perceptions of their work, and perceived knowledge needed for the work, reported a less than "rosy" picture. Of these social workers, 87 percent had MSW degrees and 11 percent had BSW degrees (Greene et al., 1992:43). Over one-half (54 percent) reported there was no more than one social worker employed by the facility (44). Staff social workers were more likely to be found in nonprofit agencies, while the consultant (part-time, contracted) social workers were more often found in proprietary facilities.

Greene and colleagues (1992) found that at least one-fourth of social workers responding to their study viewed the nursing home in which they worked as no better than minimally adequate. They rated as no better than marginal the effectiveness of their own efforts to mediate conflicts between organizational policy and resident preferences; they rated as "marginal or below" the effectiveness of the interdisciplinary team functioning. Of responding social workers, 18 percent rated their own overall effectiveness in the facility as "marginal or below" (44).

The main areas of educational/training needs identified by the social workers were categorized by Greene and colleagues (1992:48) as follows:

1. *Human behavior*—for example, knowledge of the aging process, pharmacology, neurological deficits, biopsychosocial processes, life cycle development, management of behavior of disoriented and/or aggressive patients)
2. *Methods*—for example, communication, interviewing, and intervention (especially crisis intervention and stress management, and family and group treatment interventions), time management, and data management
3. *Policy and services*—for example, entitlement programs, programs for the elderly, and OMBRA legislation
4. *Research*—for example, statistical techniques, program evaluation, and current research findings

Interdisciplinary Teamwork

That 25 percent of social worker respondents felt they were relatively ineffective on the interdisciplinary team suggests a need for improved educational preparation of health care social workers for interdisciplinary teamwork (Greene et al., 1992:52).

Cohen-Mansfield and colleagues (1991) concluded, following their study, which found some discrepancies in perceptions by nurses and social workers of patients in nursing homes, that the educational programs of both professions must provide their students with better understanding of each other's professions (146). They also concluded that the differences in professional perceptions of the status of nursing home residents' cognitive functioning, social functioning, and level of depression probably reflected differences in the skills and responsibilities of each discipline (1991:143).

Social Work Consultant Role

Social workers who wish to become employed as social work consultants to nursing homes are advised to become familiar with the state regulations (via state nursing home associations), federal guidelines, and survey procedures for nursing homes (state health departments) (Horejsi, 1987). Workshops on long-term care are also recommended, and there are books compiling examples of typical contracts and forms used (155). An assessment of the social worker designee's educational background and skills also helps to determine the kinds of help the consultant can best offer (155).

The Importance of Patient Transitioning

It is widely believed that feeling in control of one's life is positively associated with health status and sense of well-being. Therefore, social workers in health care are encouraged to support the principle of client self-determination and to avoid any and all situations and events that serve to impose unwanted, unplanned experiences on people. Thus, it is important for social workers to be aware of the types of situations or events that are high risk for such trauma to nursing home clients.

One area of needed knowledge concerns "transitioning" in and out of the nursing home. It is well established that nursing home residents often do not adapt well to sudden, forced relocation (Beirne et al., 1995). When one such facility was abruptly closed because of a temporary loss of certification for Medicaid reimbursement, a follow-up study a year later, following recertification, compared the outcome for patients who were returned within three months with those who remained elsewhere. The study found that 65 percent of those who did not return deteriorated or died, compared with 19 percent of those who returned (116). In addition, a significant difference was found in the outcome of those who had social supports and those who did not (119).

Another follow-up study (Reinardy, 1995) of elderly patients recently admitted to nursing homes found a significant positive correlation between the extent to which residents perceived that they had participated in the decision to move into the facility and their satisfaction with the facility. There was also a positive correlation between the extent to which they had wanted to move into the facility and their satisfaction with it and their level of participation in nursing home activity (36).

Scharlach (1988) found that the use of trained peer counselors, that is, other residents who reach out to newly admitted residents and provide needed information and social support, had a significant and positive effect on new residents' adaption to the facility.

Preadmission Screening for Mental Illness and Mental Retardation

Nursing home social workers responsible for resident admissions and discharges need to be aware of the following legal requirement of OMBRA 1987.

One of the many provisions of the 1987 Omnibus Budget Reconciliation Act (OMBRA) concerning nursing home reform is that patients residing in a nursing home prior to January 1, 1989 and those currently being considered for nursing home admission must undergo preadmission screening by a physician, hospital discharge planner (registered nurse or licensed social worker), or a qualified mental health and mental retardation professional. Such screenings determine whether patients have a major mental disorder or are mentally retarded or have a "related disorder," essentially another severe developmental disability (Mosher-Ashley, Turner, and O'Neill, 1991). Each state provides a standard form for such preadmission screening and resident review.

The major mental disorders of concern include schizophrenia, paranoia, major affective, schizoaffective disorders, and atypical psychoses as defined in the DSM-III (Mosher-Ashley, Turner, and O'Neill, 1991:250). The reason for the required screening is to determine which patients need professional assessment of treatment needs.

This concern over mental disorders arose as a result of the deinstitutionalization movement since the 1950s, which resulted in large numbers of transfers of institutionalized mentally ill and developmentally disabled persons from state hospitals into Medicaid-certified nursing homes, where, for the most part, the services they needed were not available. OMBRA requires that any such patients who do not need nursing home care must be relocated to a more appropriate setting, unless they have resided in the facility for thirty months or more and wish to stay (Mosher-Ashley, Turner, and O'Neill, 1991:250).

Nursing Home Ombudsman Program

Nursing home social workers should be aware that since Congress created the Long-Term Care Ombudsman Program in 1978 under the Older Americans Act, most states have such a program. States have the option of employing people to fill these positions or using volunteers. The effectiveness of these programs varies considerably, but reviewers of such programs have generally agreed that the best ombudsman programs attract, train, and retain volunteers (Nelson, 1995). The 1987 Older Americans Act strengthened the authority and responsibility of ombudsmen, assuring them access to nursing home facilities, and many states specify such responsibilities as complaint investigation, technical assistance and training, advocacy with coordination with other state agencies, public education, and program management and development (Nelson, 1995:32). Some of the features of more effective ombudsman programs include high visibility, rapid handling of complaints, legal support, independent status, and strong enabling legislation (36). As one ombudsman reported:

> . . . when we walk in, the staff starts hopping. They are very aware of who we are and why we're there. It's hard to know for sure, but they feel my presence there. The administration and staff are much more attentive to the care and dignity of the residents. (Nelson, 1995:39)

VALUES AND ETHICS CONSIDERATIONS

Legitimate Sources of Patient Information

There are multiple and complex values and ethics issues of which nursing home social workers ought to be cognizant. One of these is that using family or staff "proxies" for information concerning residents is hazardous because some evidence suggests that such alternate informants may not know as much about the residents as is sometimes assumed (Tennstedt et al., 1992).

Residents' Rights and Proactive Care Preferences

Since the Patient Self-Determination Act of 1990, one of the many functions usually assigned to the social worker in a nursing home is to inform each resident soon after admission, or a family member if the patient appears incompetent, of the *patient rights* in the facility. Then the social worker should explore with residents their specific wishes concerning medical decisions and determine whether they have, or are interested in having, a "durable power of attorney" and a "living will." Most nursing homes have written documents to assist in this process and usually try to obtain *a living will* (signed statement, witnessed by two people, clarifying the residents wishes about the circumstances under which they do or do not wish to be provided with medical treatment, nutrition and hydration, and pain medication).

A *durable power of attorney* is a legal document that must be completed while the person is still mentally competent. This document allocates responsibility to a specified other to make specific kinds of decisions on the person's behalf should he or she become incompetent to act alone. The person is expected to discuss with the designee or agent what he or she wishes done in the future, given certain circumstances, and the agent is expected to honor those wishes.

Needless to say, discussing issues of future disability and death with nursing home residents and their families requires considerable sensitivity to their feelings. Newly admitted patients and their families are understandably anxious and often overwhelmed with simply adjusting to all the change and uncertainty associated with nursing home admission. Thus, the social worker ought to individualize each situation in terms of deciding when the most opportune and appropriate occasion is to attempt to engage residents and/or families in considering these serious issues.

Nonetheless, they need to be discussed soon, for the following reason:

> The absence of advance directives can lead to stress, confusion, painful introspection, and expenditure of time and emotional and financial resources by both family members and health care providers who are forced to exert a substituted judgement. (Spears, Drinka, and Voeks, 1993:409)

In cases in which the client is already incompetent to either select a power of attorney or to make advance directives, legal action to appoint a guardian may be necessary (Spears, Drinka, and Voeks, 1993:409). State laws may vary concerning these alternate procedures so social workers need to become familiar with those in their particular states.

The Issue of Resident Autonomy

Social workers who wish to work in nursing home-type settings would do well to obtain a copy of an excellent book concerning ethical dilemmas in nursing homes, edited by Kane and Caplan (1990). It could serve as an ongoing reference source in helping to resolve ethical issues and be used for in-service training with nursing home staff. Underlying position in this book is as follows:

> The mission of the nursing home must be to assist residents in their attempts to exercise their autonomous will rather than to manage their behavior. Resident autonomy for all residents capable of asserting it must replace institutional efficiency as the central goal. . . . (Foldes, 1990:35)

The issue of autonomy or self-determination is closely related to quality of life. It is not enough that nursing home patients are allowed to designate a durable power of attorney or complete a living will; it is all the little decisions of everyday life that make the difference in an individual's sense of control, which is vital to happiness, health, and well-being. People need to decide for themselves when they will get up in the morning and go to bed at night, when they will eat and what they will eat, when they need to go to the toilet, what they will wear, and which activities they will engage in (Caplan, 1990:39-41).

The principle of respect for autonomy implies *individualized care* in the nursing home setting (Kane and Caplan, 1990:81) and requires that staff really know their residents' likes and dislikes, values, beliefs, habits, behavioral patterns, and so forth.

The Death and Dying of Residents

Another area of nursing home care that is often dealt with poorly is the death of a resident. Most residents and their families need and want to know what is going on and to have death and dying dealt with honestly and respectfully. Both the dying resident and his or home that they cannot expose their vulnerability enough to share their innermost feelings of sadness.

Addressing the Hostile-Aggressive Nursing Home Resident

Cox (1993) reminds us that the primary goal of social work is to improve the functioning of the person in his or her environmental context. Therefore, it is inappropriate to assume that the cause of hostile-aggressive behavior of a nursing home resident is entirely intrapsychic and to attempt to deal with it through chemical and/or physical restraints.

Instead, Cox (1993) recommends a behavioral assessment to search for underlying contributing conditions, such as hearing or speech impairments; organic brain syndrome; interpersonal relationships with staff, roommate, and family; recent history of losses; and impact of nursing home rules, regulations, activities, and restrictions on resident autonomy.

Cox (1993) points out that aggressive behavior is often a natural response to feeling threatened and, in some ways, may be a healthier alternative to "giving up" and subsequent withdrawal and depression, however dysfunctional for the facility. Thus, the social worker is expected to mediate between the needs of the resident and those of the nursing home operation.

Depending on the identified causes of the disruptive behavior, interventions may include supportive therapy and counseling, behavioral approaches, environmental change, operant conditioning, reality orientation, physical restraints, and medications (Cox, 1993:186). Cox (1993) discusses each type of intervention and cites examples of appropriate circumstances of their use (186-190):

1. Supportive therapy—including group therapy, can help with problems associated with adjusting to the nursing home placement. The focus is on expression of feelings and receiving emotional support from others to build a sense of competency to cope.

2. Behavioral approaches—involve identifying the antecedents of the behavior that needs changing and learning a new response to it, such as relaxation techniques or assertiveness training to express thoughts and feelings without provoking the other person.

3. Environmental change—may involve changing roommates, advocating for more staff accommodation to resident preferences, inducing involvement in activities and/or social interaction, and in-service training to improve staff understanding of, and sensitivity to, resident needs.

4. *Operant conditioning*—involves the use of positive responses (rewards) or negative responses (loss of enjoyed things) to induce desired behavior. The behavior and the response must be consistently and immediately combined so that the person is "reconditioned" or "retaught." Positive reinforcement is generally preferred, both for humanitarian reasons and because it has the advantage of reinforcing the desired behavior rather than simply discouraging the undesirable behavior.

5. *Reality orientation*—is used with residents who are temporarily confused and agitated because of too much environmental change and stimuli, sometimes combined with early cognitive frailty. This approach can involve maintaining a calm, consistent routine with a lack of stimulation; reminders of the date, day, and time from family and staff; and a constantly warm and reassuring manner that both models the desired behavior and calms the resident. Calendars, clocks, photographs, and familiar objects can be helpful with this approach.

6. *Physical and chemical restraints*—are generally discouraged, having been found to be both physically and psychologically damaging. Since OMBRA 1987, severe restrictions are placed on nursing homes in their ability to use either form of restraint. Social workers should never be party to their use and are required to take action to prevent their use, except temporarily, in a dire emergency and with the order of a physician. Physical restraints are now believed to be associated with increased risk of injury from falls out of bed (Evans and Strumpf, 1989, cited in Bruno, 1994:139), abnormal changes in body chemistry, increased basal metabolic rate and blood volume, orthostatic hypotension, contractures, lower extremity edema and decubitus ulcers, decreased muscle mass and tone/strength, bone demineralization, overgrowth of opportunistic organisms, and EEG (electroencephalogram) changes (Evans and Strumpf, 1989, cited in Bruno, 1994:132).

In addition, restraints can lead to disorganized behavior, emotional desolation, fear of abandonment, feelings of being punished, sensory deprivation, and loss of self-esteem (Bruno, 1994:132). Bruno (1994), citing Williams (1989:585), wrote:

The key to restraint free care . . . is to practice "individualized care," centered on the person, and his or her particular
needs . . . staff must get to know the resident, not merely as a
"patient" . . . and they need to continue to work together to
exchange information and ideas. (141)

Another social worker (Lerer, 1995) employed in a veterans'
extended care facility reported on her experience working with the
"irascible" patient. She observed that most of the facility's predominately male patients "have a strong sense of entitlement" (171) as
veterans and tend to be cognitively intact, but severely impaired
physically, often nonambulatory, and incontinent. In addition, they
often have a lack of impulse control and a history of lack of lasting
social relationships. Lerer (1995) expressed her belief that the
physical dependency of these patients produces low self-esteem and
acting-out behavior (172), which reflects a sort of regression to an
earlier developmental stage (173).

Lerer (1995) has described her counseling with such patients,
which involves an "initial stage" of attentive listening to ventilation
of complaints, offering support and acceptance, and modeling patient, calm behavior. In a "middle stage," she explored with the
patient his background history, interests, and hobbies, as well as his
ideas about what would constitute "ideal" care from the staff. The
understanding and acceptance from the worker gradually calms the
patient, who begins to get in touch with his innermost feelings of
loneliness and despair. He remembers "who he was," before his
physical impairment and adult dependency, and this helps to restore
his self-esteem. In the "sustaining stage," the patient begins to grieve
his losses, to improve his self-esteem, and to be less depressed.
Relationships with other staff improve, and the social worker provides less frequent, but ongoing, emotional and social support. The
worker lets the nursing staff know how they have helped the social
worker to better understand that the patient's abusive behavior is his
response to his fear and sense of loss of control (Lerer, 1995:78).
In-service training by the social worker with online staff is an important supplement to more effectively dealing with "irascible" patients, through a combination of teaching, opportunity for ventilation, exchange of concerns and ideas, and mutual support.

Dealing with Aggressive Members of Residents' Families

A less familiar problem in nursing homes is that of family members who reportedly are rude and otherwise verbally abusive toward staff, largely in reaction to what they perceive as poor care of their resident loved ones. A survey (Vinton and Mazza, 1994) of seventy nursing homes in Florida obtained reports of more than one thousand acts of verbal aggression and thirteen acts of physical aggression on the part of residents' family members toward nursing home care staff during a six-month period.

Daughters (31 percent) and wives (28 percent) were more often reported as the aggressors than were husbands (14 percent) or sons (11 percent), and the rest (16 percent) were perpetrated by a variety of other relatives (Vinton and Mazza, 1994:530). Social work staff were reported to be the ones most often asked to resolve such conflicts, and Vinton and Mazza (1994) comment that since most of the conflicts concerned an issue related to the quality of nursing service, one wonders why they were not most often resolved by the nursing directors.

The strategies most often used to resolve such conflicts were reported to be (1) discussing the situation with the staff person, (2) discussing the situation with the aggressive family member, and (3) discussing the situation with the staff person and family member together. Vinton and Mazza (1994) note that since other possible alternative approaches listed on the questionnaire—such as in-service training, using the resident's care plan for care criteria, establishing policy, and contracting with family members—were not used, many potential avenues for conflict resolution are not being explored by nursing home social workers and others who are asked to address such problem situations.

Another study (Wullschleger et al., 1996), a nationwide survey of family caregivers who were members of caregiver support groups, found that those whose care recipient relative was now in a nursing home had the highest measured level of anxiety about their own anticipated aging. It was not clear whether this resulted from a fear of deterioration or from fear of themselves becoming recipients of poor-quality care in such facilities. However, the reportedly heightened anxiety about their own future aging may help to explain some of the aggressive behavior of family members toward nursing home staff, as reported in other studies.

Helping Former Family Caregivers

As the previous paragraph suggests, family members who were home care caregivers of the nursing home resident before the placement may have special difficulty adjusting to the placement (Montgomery and Kosloski, 1994; Riddick et al., 1992).

According to Riddick and colleagues (1992):

> While admission to a nursing home may diminish the amount of time a (family) caregiver needs to devote daily to his/her loved one, other concerns apparently arise and consume the attention of the caregiver. More specifically, the caregiver still experiences burdens surrounding the caregiver role, and emotional conflicts over his/her relative's placement in the nursing home. (70-71)

In addition, family caregivers often have devoted a significant period of their lives in the caregiving role prior to their loved ones' placement. Riddick and colleagues (1992) found the average length of time was seven years (58), and satisfaction with the nursing home was inversely related to the family caregiver's ongoing sense of burden following the placement.

Caregiver burden refers to the family caregiver's sense of internal conflict concerning such emotions as unhappiness, guilt, anger, depression, and anxiety over one's future (Riddick et al., 1992:52). Monahan (1995) called it "felt stress" and pointed out that some observers have suggested that it may even increase after institutional placement. Riddick and colleagues (1992) report what one daughter said of her feelings about placing her parent with dementia in a nursing home:

> [I realize that] I must somehow "learn" I must be responsible for myself first or I'll die. Intellectually, I know the answer, but it is very difficult to carry out. How do you abandon those you love? (72)

According to Riddick and colleagues (1992), the practice implications are that social workers must (1) provide family caregivers with counseling that addresses the emotions they tend to experience both before and following the placement; (2) educate them concerning nursing home life; (3) sensitize nursing home staff to what the family caregivers experience; and (4) teach nursing home staff behaviors that facilitate the residents' and families' adjustment and acceptance of the nursing home—especially spouses of residents, who have greater difficulty relinquishing their former role to the staff (72).

That former family caregivers continue to feel responsible monitoring the nursing home care of their loved ones is suggested by the finding of Dempsey and Pruchno (1993) that the tasks assumed by family caregivers after the placement reflect the "principle of substitution." That is, family caregivers tend to assume whatever tasks they perceive the residents need done that the staff have not covered, especially nontechnical ones (141).

Dempsey and Pruchno (1993) recommend the following: (1) family caregivers need to understand which tasks the nursing home should be responsible for providing (mostly technical tasks, such as toileting, bathing, dressing, feeding, administering medicines and treatments); (2) nursing home staff should be encouraged to view the family caregivers as competent to assist in the residents' care, especially in the provision of nontechnical services (such as managing their money, shopping, providing plants and other "extras" in the room, marking the residents identification on their clothing and other possessions, giving or withholding consent for procedures, and writing letters); and (3) staff should help family caregivers to find activities they can share during visits to relieve family members' sense of helplessness (143).

Monahan (1995) reported the findings of a survey of former family caregivers of patients admitted to a dementia unit in a nursing home in New York in an effort to identify variables associated with the level of "caregiver burden." The variables that best explained the variance in caregiver burden were caregiver health (poorer health equaled greater burden); age and gender (older and male caregivers felt more burdened); race, marital status, and educational level (nonwhites, married, and those with higher educational levels had more burden); and caregiver perception of the quality of nursing home care (the poorer the perceived quality, the greater the burden). Monahan (1995) also recommends that social workers in nursing homes help family caregivers and staff to develop "partnerships for care planning and provision" to avoid staff interpretations of family "overinvolvement" and to help reduce family caregiver burden.

COMMENTARY

Clearly, there is a need to design a system for nursing home care reimbursement that serves to promote a higher quality of care, both in terms of medical services as well as personal care services, with an overriding incentive to rehabilitate rather than merely "warehouse." Nursing home care needs to be designed to fulfill, in practice, the theoretical concept of caring at the third stage of the care continuum: rehabilitation and maximization of comfort and function.

People should not have to impoverish themselves to be able to pay for nursing home care through Medicaid. Long-term care needs to be a Medicare provision, regardless of care level, so that people who need the services are not humiliated by economic dependency in addition to dealing with care dependency.

Health and social services must be nonprofit if they are to have quality care as their primary objective. It is obscene to reduce nursing home care, or any other health or social service, to a business enterprise. Of course, if home care were made more feasible, economically and otherwise, nursing home care could be reduced.

Quality nonprofit facilities could doubtlessly use some of the savings from what formerly went to stockholders to provide better training, pay, and benefits to the certified nursing assistant (CNA) staff, thereby improving the quality of services and reducing online staff turnover. In addition, CNA staff need to be included in ID team meetings, since they are the ones who work most closely with the patients.

Patients themselves need to be engaged in future redesign of the structure and program of nursing homes. This would not only help to empower the residents, thereby facilitating their potential well-being, but also provide for adapting the environment to residents' cultural needs, health condition needs, and personal preferences. Presumably, any organization in which the "customers" are satisfied and truly "like" the service is likely to be a happier place for staff as well. As the data indicate, in nursing homes, this apparently is a function of staff and resident empowerment.

Clearly, many nursing home facilities do not employ enough social workers with the needed training and skills to adequately address residents' needs or meet NASW standards for social work services in nursing homes. This is due, to a great extent, to the for-profit status of most nursing homes in the United States. As we have seen in our presentation of social work services in other health care settings, the numbers and degree level of social work staff tend to be inversely associated with the profit orientation of the facility. After all, it is far cheaper to employ someone "on call" than full-time, to hire one person when you need two or three, and to select someone with a BSW rather than an MSW. The problem is that if you actually need one or more such people full-time, and the problems you want them to address are not something those with BSWs are qualified to do, questions arise about the adequacy of the care provided.

Finally, hopefully, everyone would agree that family caregivers and other loved ones should not have to feel that they are sending their relatives to a "house of horrors," if not to their deaths, when they finally realize that they simply must admit their loved ones to a nursing home, nor should anyone live their later lives with the fear that such may be their own end.

Chapter 7

Social Work in Hospice Care

HISTORICAL BACKGROUND

The terms hospice, hospital, hotel, and hostel imply "hosting" or providing hospitality, that is, warmly receiving and taking care of the needs of one's fellow human beings. Hospice care emerged in the 300s A.D. in the region of the Holy Land through the efforts of the Eastern Orthodox Christian Church, as a means of offering aid to needy travelers, often going to or coming from religious sites (Kerr, 1993:2). A well-to-do Roman woman, Fabiola, witnessed such care by the Eastern Church and carried the idea back to Italy, where she and a Roman senator, Pammachius, began a similar program in Ostia, a Mediterranean port city (Phipps, 1988).

In the fifth century, St. Bridget of Ireland established what amounted to a hospice for ill or dying people (Richman, 1995:1358). During the Middle Ages, religious orders often opened their doors to travelers in need—such as poor, ill, disabled, and dying persons—and called their service a "hospice" or "hostel" (Proffitt, 1987:813).

In 1846, a Catholic Mother and founder of the Irish Sisters of Charity, Sister Mary Aikenhead, opened her home in Dublin, Ireland, to care for the dying. After her death, her Daughters in Christ, in response to her example and inspiration, established Our Lady's Hospice (Richman, 1995:1359-1364; Kerr, 1993:13).

In the late 1800s, in the United States, the Dominican Sisters began to provide inpatient care of dying persons, following the English pattern, and their programs continue today (Proffitt, 1987:813). In 1905, the idea of hospice care caught hold in London, and St. Joseph's Hospice was established. A medical social worker and nurse, Cicely Saunders, later worked there and eventually became a physician (Richman, 1995:1359). In 1967, at age fifty-seven, Saunders opened another hospice, called St. Christopher's of London, which became a famous center for research and teaching concerning the care of dying people, as well as a model for quality hospice care services, both inpatient and at home (Richman, 1995:1359; Kron, 1978). St. Christopher's Hospice was the site of great advances in pain management through the work of Saunders, and her work ignited the modern hospice movement (Proffitt, 1987:813).

Modeled after St. Christopher's, the Hospice of Connecticut, in New Haven, was established in the United States in 1974 (Hayslip and Leon, 1992; McNulty and Holderby, 1983; Paradis, 1985; Saunders, 1982). However, in the United States, the concept of hospice care soon developed into a specific care philosophy, with its associated program of services, apart from a particular "place." Whereas the European hospice model revolved around palliative care in a facility known as a "hospice," in America, hospice care became a home care-based program. In October 1983, hospice programs were approved by Medicare to provide continued care, whatever setting the patient entered (National Association for Home Care, 1996).

Growth and Cost of Hospice Care

Medicare

In 1985, the first year when Medicare payments were made for hospice services, 43 million dollars were so spent but during 1994, a total of 1 billion, 486 million dollars in Medicare payments was expended for hospice care (U.S. Government Printing Office, 1995:115), indicating about an 11.3-fold increase during the first ten-year period of Medicare coverage. Still, in 1995, only about 1 percent of total Medicare benefit payments for all types of health care services were for hospice care (National Association for Home Care, 1996).

Medicaid

"Hospice is an optional Medicaid benefit which is currently offered by 38 states. Payments for hospice services were estimated at $198 million in FY94" (National Association for Home Care, 1996:6). This amount represented only two-tenths of 1 percent of total Medicaid expenditures.

Other Payers

Presumably, an additional significant amount of hospice care is paid for out of pocket, since a large percentage of hospice-providing organizations are not certified by any standard-setting organization.

THEORETICAL PERSPECTIVES

The Concept of Caring

As its history suggests, hospice care is a moral imperative, rooted in the value of concern about human suffering and the ethical sense of responsibility to help relieve that suffering. As Eric Cassell (1982) pointed out, suffering is caused not only by physical pain, but also by the sense that personal integrity is endangered.

As the medical profession developed a curative technology and associated value system during the twentieth century, physicians grew to regard chronic and terminal health problems as personal failures and to withdraw from such situations with the attitude, and sometimes the remark, that "nothing more can be done" (Preston, 1979). Such a stance reflects a lack of recognition that even when people are terminally ill, they still have other needs while they are alive—such as relief from suffering—whether biological, psychological, social, or spiritual. Such relief of suffering is referred to as *palliative care*, meaning "comfort care."

The difference between the medical model and the hospice model and the difficulties of introducing a hospice service within a traditional health care setting are elaborated by Wade Smith (1994). He notes that the adjustment is not only a shift away from the focus on curing but also a shift from technology to the use of interpersonal relationship as the principle healing force, something in which physicians are not as well trained (204-206). Freund and McGuire (1991) add that contemporary biomedicine is essentially directed toward the conquest of death, and even though it cannot always cure disease, it, unfortunately, often can prolong life. This reflects the *technological imperative*, that is, the compulsion to employ a technology if it is available (253-254).

The objective of hospice care is to maximize the quality of a patient's remaining life and to facilitate his or her "safe passage." According to Corbett and Hai (1979), the objective of hospice care is "euthanatos," or a "good death," that is, a death preceded by intensive *caring* rather than intensive care. Hospice care does not substitute for family care, but rather supplements and supports family care as needed. The units of care and attention in the hospice philosophy are the patient, family, and caregiving staff (Rusnack, Schaefer, and Moxley, 1988), and hospice care is conceptualized as escorting the patient in his or her transition to death, during which caregivers keep company with the dying to ensure a safe passage (Corr and Corr, 1985).

Essentially, the hospice perspective is one of *caring* at the tertiary level of health services, that is, giving supportive assistance to maximize comfort and function and to prevent secondary disabilities from lack of appropriate societal responses to a primary impairment. This can be accomplished through providing needed services, tools and equipment, income supports, environmental modifications, and supportive interpersonal interactions. Caring, in whatever form, revolves around *empowering* the person, that is, strengthening his or her sense of wholeness, intactness, and control. Thus, the patient must be personalized and individualized with a strong supportive relationship.

Biopsychosocial and Holistic Perspectives

The motivation to provide hospice care is essentially an ethical one. The interventions provided by hospice workers emerge from a developing body of theory and knowledge about such issues as the nature of suffering and the control of pain; healthy and unhealthy grief and bereavement; the interaction and interdependence of mind, body, social and cultural environments, and spiritual needs;

the family as a system; and the etiology and modification of a person's sense of *locus of control.*

Hospice care has a *holistic* perspective in that it directs attention to the needs of the whole person. In an inspirational keynote address, Balfour Mount (1993), physician and director of Palliative Care at McGill University in Montreal, talked about whole-person care as involving interaction with the "spiritual" person of the patient as well as attending to his or her physical needs. Mount describes *spiritual* as that part of a person capable of transcendence (34).

Hospice care has a *biopsychosocial* perspective, recognizing that the biological, psychological, and social spheres of our lives interact and affect one another. We use the term *social* to include not only relationships and interactions with other people through family, groups, organizations, community, and society but also cultural influences, such as ethnicity, language, values and beliefs, customs and traditions, social status, and religion or spirituality. Hospice health care professionals know that the experience of physical pain is greater when the patient is feeling hungry, lonely, guilty, remorseful, afraid, powerless, ashamed, unfit, misunderstood, rejected, or abandoned (Strang, 1992; Mount, 1993:28).

Continuity of Care

Because terminally ill people often reside in a variety of settings during their passage from assessment of terminal status to death—including hospital, home, and nursing home—the hospice philosophy also includes the importance of ensuring "continuity of care." As a program rather than a place, hospice care can follow the patient from setting to setting, and hospice philosophy holds that it is necessary to do so to ensure ongoing quality of comfort care.

Primary Prevention

In a sense, hospice care is not only a form of tertiary care but also a form of primary preventive care. Its inclusion of bereavement care for the family, which continues after the patient's death serves to help reduce the potential impact of the stress of unresolved grief on family members' health and life expectancy (Stubblefield, 1990).

Hospice philosophy recognizes that loved ones who will be left behind need to have time and opportunity to express their grief so they can go on with their own lives afterward with maximum well-being. In fact, stress research indicates that unresolved grief is a significant factor in predicting health status and life expectancy (Weiner, 1984:258).

Systems Perspective

Hospice programs, and social work performed within them, also have a *systems perspective* in the sense of recognizing the inter-dependence of biological, psychological, and social systems as well as that of the various levels of social organization: individual, family, small group, organization, community, and society. That is, the effectiveness of the hospice program itself depends in part on the patient's family; the hospice organization's structure, auspice, and philosophy; the resources available from other community organizations; and the social welfare policies and programs enabled by the society's economic and political systems. In short, how we live and how we die is not entirely up to us, but is influenced by all the social structures in our environment on which we are interdependent.

HUMAN DIVERSITY RELEVANCE

In discussing the social worker's psychosocial assessment of the hospice patient and family, Lusk (1983) wrote: "To be responsive to the uniqueness of each patient-family system, the social history must be cognizant of ethnic and cultural considerations" (213). This is especially necessary given the significant variations across nationalities, religions, ethnicities, sexual orientation, and gender regarding attitudes and practices relating to death and dying. It is important for hospice workers to be aware of these variations and to know where to look to learn about clients' unfamiliar culture. A major and recent resource for this type of information is the text edited by Parry and Ryan (1995). A list of other related resources may be found at the end of this chapter.

As indicated earlier in this book, variation exists both between groups and within groups, so one cannot assume that because a person is a member of a certain group that he or she holds a certain set of values, beliefs, customs, and so on. Again, social workers need to be familiar with the client's general group culture, but also should explore with the individual how his or her own convictions do or do not conform to those of the group.

Some of the ways in which cultural variations can influence appropriate hospice care include the following:

- Customs concerning whether to tell the person (and his or her family) that the condition is terminal
- Attitudes toward the use of various types of medicines, both traditional and folk medicines (for example, many cultures have prohibitions against the extensive use of opiates to control pain)
- Perceptions of what sort of physical environment would be peaceful, beautiful, comfortable, and so on
- Religious implications for encouraging the client and/or family to express anxieties, concerns, questions, feelings of guilt, and so forth
- Attitudes concerning efforts to prolong life and/or to facilitate death when a person is in severe pain and death is inevitable

In short, human diversity variables may affect perspectives on practically everything: appropriate clothing, food, conversation, and pain relief; the meaning of death and the allocation of roles; disposition of the deceased's body; bereavement practices; the significance of certain colors; dying at home; and the extent to which patient, family, and health care providers should be involved in decision making (Parry and Ryan, 1995; Storey, 1993).

INTERDISCIPLINARY TEAMWORK

Concept of Interdisciplinary Teamwork

Interdisciplinary teamwork differs from multidisciplinary teamwork in that team members are not simply all attending to the same "case," but are cooperating in and coordinating their work, that is, operating together toward the same end.

Rationale for Interdisciplinary Teamwork

Because hospice care recognizes the interaction of biological, psychological, and social factors, it adopts a team approach. The team can include the family, supervising physician, nurses, nursing assistants, social worker, chaplain, physical therapist, occupational therapist, and so forth, as needed, with members cooperating in a type of "group practice."

Medicare Standards for Hospice Team Composition

Medicare standards for hospice programs name the core members of the interdisciplinary team as including at least "a doctor of medicine or osteopathy, registered nurse, social worker, and a pastoral or other counselor," with other professionals added as needed (U.S. Government Printing Office, 1994:26).

The National Hospice Organization Recommendation for Hospice Team Composition

The National Hospice Organization suggests that the core group needed to provide quality hospice service should include the patient's attending physician, registered nurses, clergy or other spiritual counselor, master's-level social workers, and trained volunteers (Richman, 1995:1360-1361). Note that this differs from the Medicare standard by specifying the need for both MSWs and trained volunteers.

The Effect of Per Diem Reimbursement on Team Composition

A current problem with Medicare's per diem reimbursement for hospice care is that the hospice organization, whether public, proprietary, or voluntary, must decide which services it can afford to provide for the set daily fee. This may require settling for less than optimum team composition and services.

The Dilemma of Role Flexibility Without Role Subsumption

Because not all team members are with the patient all the time, roles need to be flexible. This can be a strength of hospice teamwork, but also can be a source of tension and role ambiguity (McDonald, 1991:276; Kulys and Davis, 1986; Donovan, 1984).

According to Fish (1994:411), role overlap or blurring is inevitable. A potential problem is that those professionals who are required to be with the patient the most, such as the nurses, may be inclined to assume the functions of other team members, for example, providing psychosocial assessment and counseling or acting as a liaison with other community agencies, which are the responsibilities the social worker. This can lead to the latter being used less and less often and eventually being excluded from the core team altogether (Dush, 1988a). At the same time, the staff person who assumes the functions of others becomes burdened with excessive demands, and the patient and family receive lower-quality service because of the difference in training and experience in that particular function.

Rodway and Blythe (1994) commented:

> While there are many advantages to a team approach to palliative care, the lack of a clearly delineated model of palliative care may well be the result of its interdisciplinary nature. (421)

ORGANIZATIONAL CONSIDERATIONS

The same kinds of organizational considerations affecting social work practice in other health service settings also influence hospice social work.

Organizational Ownership

For example, whether the organization is public, private nonprofit, or private for profit will be a determinant of organizational goals and objectives. According to the 1994 National Home and Hospice Care Survey, 90.4 percent of hospice organizations were voluntary nonprofit, 7.3 percent were proprietary, and 2.3 percent were government and other types of organizations (U.S. Government Printing Office, 1995:135).

When the major goal of the health service organization is financial profit for shareholders rather than delivering the highest possible quality of human health services to its clients, and unless specific quantities and qualities of services are mandated by standard-setting organizations, the incentive is to reduce service quality and quantity to whatever level will enhance profit margins. Oftentimes, this results in the employment of too few staff, with minimal rather than optimal qualifications, to do the work, and "soft" services whose impact is apt to be measurable only qualitatively, such as social work and clergy, are likely to be minimally provided. Reductions in staff size and qualifications imply a reduction in the amount and quality of client care services.

Sectarian or Secular

Whether the organization is sectarian or secular and the nature of the religious beliefs of a sectarian organization will influence professional practice in the hospice setting.

Governing Standards

The rules and regulations of the funding sources concerning client eligibility for service also make a difference, such as whether a family caregiver must be present or whether reimbursement for services is per diem, per capita, or fee for service. Again, per diem or per capita structures reduce costs through reducing services.

Certification Status

Another organizational variable of interest is whether the agency providing hospice services is "certified." In 1995, there were 1,857 Medicare-certified hospice agencies in the United States. In addition, about 1,974, or 25 percent, of the 7,897 noncertified home care agencies in the United States were providing primarily hospice services, bringing the total to about 3,831 hospice agencies, of which only about 48.5 percent were Medicare certified (National Association for Home Care, 1996). Currently, Medicare is the only standard-setting mechanism for hospices with any authority (Sontag, 1996).

Somewhat different data are found on hospice certification in *Statistical Abstracts of the United States* (U.S. Government Printing Office, 1995:135), which indicates that in 1994, 69.2 percent of hospice-providing organizations were Medicare certified and 59.9 percent were Medicaid certified. These data are also reported to be derived from the 1994 National Home and Hospice Care Survey.

In late 1993 and early 1994, Sontag (1996) studied a stratified random sample of U.S. hospice programs and found, among other things, that the Medicare-certified programs sought such certification primarily to enhance their credibility, and hence income, and were more likely than non-Medicare-certified hospices to focus on the medical problems of patients and to use more professional and fewer volunteer staff. In addition, a higher percentage of staff of noncertified hospice programs reported high staff morale. Finally, Medicare-certified hospices were more likely to require patients to sign a "do not resuscitate" (DNR) order and less likely to require a family primary caregiver (PCG) before accepting them into their programs (37-40).

Sontag (1996) also found that Medicare-certified hospices were more likely to be affiliated with a medical service organization, such as a hospital or home care agency, and thus may be more entrapped in the traditional "medical model." If so, there may be less attention to psychosocial needs of patients and families, generally provided by master's-level social workers with training in assessment and counseling of such needs, and other staff may sense the negative effects of such a lack on the patients and their families, thereby eroding employee morale.

With the increase in certification by Medicare and in affiliation with medical care organizations rather than freestanding voluntary organizations, hospice programs also have begun to employ a variety of "technology" types (Kaye and Davitt, 1995:263). Some of this technology raises a question about whether the pure philosophy of hospice care is being contaminated by the traditional health care sector—and its "medical model."

CLIENT PROBLEMS
AND SOCIAL WORKER FUNCTIONS

Introduction

As has been pointed out, hospice is a program and a philosophy rather than a particular place or setting. However, although most hospice care is provided in the home, hospice agencies sometimes follow former home care patients into nursing homes to provide continuity of appropriate care. In addition, acute care hospitals sometimes provide hospice care service on the hospital site—partly as a result of the trend in hospitals toward vertical integration of health care services other than acute care, as acute-care stays are shortened by cost-saving government measures. Furthermore, there are some freestanding hospice facilities in the United States especially for AIDS patients. Thus, client problems and social worker functions relating to hospice care are made more complex by the variation in type of organizational setting.

Client Problems

From the perspective of social worker functions, the problems of patients in hospice care may be classified as those associated with (1) admission to the hospice service; (2) adjustment to the service or facility; (3) adjustment to the diagnosis, prognosis, or care plan; (4) the lack of information to make informed decisions and take control; and (5) the lack of needed supportive resources, such as supportive tools and equipment, support services, income supports, supportive environmental adaptations, and interpersonal supports; and (6) barriers to discharge from the service or setting.

Barriers to Admission

Terminally ill patients and their families often need someone to help assess their financial resources and eligibility for coverage under the various available sources of funding for hospice care. In addition, they may need help in coming to terms with the diagnosis, prognosis, and recommended care plan; for example, acceptance of Medicare coverage for hospice care requires an agreement that all curative efforts will cease in favor of palliative care. This coming-to-terms process often involves working through questions they may have and providing information to help address those issues. Finally, terminally ill patients and/or their families may have practical issues—such as how family members will manage financially if they take a leave of absence from their employment to help care for the patient or who will stay with the patient while the family care-giver goes shopping or simply "gets away" every now and then.

Adjustment to the Service or Facility

Much hospice care is provided in the patient's home by a home care agency. Having "outsiders" coming and going is a major adjustment for most people. Some concerns may be about staff stealing from the home, failing to secure locks on doors when they leave, or simply invading the family's privacy. Most people are accustomed to feeling relatively independent, especially in their own home. Consequently, home hospice care can produce conflicting feelings of both gratitude for the help and resentment regarding the sense of helplessness and dependency.

If patients are to be admitted to a hospice facility, whether freestanding or within a nursing home or hospital unit, the idea of being in "a place to die" can seem threatening. Most people feel more vulnerable in such a facility than they would in their own homes. On the other hand, the social worker can help by pointing out the advantages of such places. For example, some hospice sites may offer the assurance of more effective pain control, supervision by qualified professionals, ready access to oxygen to ease breathing distress, high standards of cleanliness, and ever-present staff to assist when needed. Further, some terminally ill patients may find it comforting to interact with other terminally ill people and to share with others a common experience, especially if the facility promotes a "homey" atmosphere, one, for example, that permits patients to keep pets or to have wine with their dinner, if they wish.

Adjustment to the Diagnosis, Prognosis, or Care Plan

Coming to terms with a serious diagnosis, especially one that is imminently terminal, is usually experienced as gravely threatening. This process involves dealing with many complex feelings and questions. Aside from the terminal prognosis, the diagnosis itself sometimes raises issues concerning the expected effect on physical attractiveness, the possible judgments of other people regarding the etiology of the disorder and the patient's previous lifestyle, preconceptions about ultimate pain and suffering, and how loved ones will cope with the diagnosis.

As is now well known, awareness of impending death, either one's own or a loved one's, is experienced as a loss to be grieved.

The grief experience is thought to pass through a series of stages, varying in order among different people, but generally including such responses as denial, anger, bargaining. depression, and acceptance or resignation (Kübler-Ross, 1969).

Adjustment to the recommended care plan concerns issues such as trading further curative efforts for comfort care and coming to terms with site and/or provider selection among the available options.

Lack of Information to Make Informed Decisions and Feel in Control

Terminally ill patients are particularly prone to a sense of diminished control. The social worker, with other team members, plays a vital role in helping patients and their families to counteract this tendency by providing them with honest and accurate answers to their questions, as well as relevant information to assist them in thinking through their decisions.

Lack of Resources to Meet Needs

In the role of case manager, the social worker is often responsible for, and best suited to, ascertaining the clients' resource needs from talking with them, family members, and other team staff and to assist them in obtaining such resources. Resource needs vary, not only with client and family situation, but also with the hospice care setting. However, most patients are cared for at home and are not likely to own equipment such as a hospital bed, bedside commode, suction machine, Hoya lift, portable oxygen, and so on. Needed resources can include medical aids and appliances/tools and equipment, supplemental services, income supports, environmental adaptations, and interpersonal supports.

Barriers to Discharge

Discharge planning refers to assisting the patient and family in making arrangements for termination of one service and transfer to another setting and/or service. In the case of hospice care, patient service is usually terminated upon death. However, most hospice programs provide varying amounts of bereavement care service to the family following a patient's death. Presumably, some family members may become quite attached to hospice staff, and either or both may find it difficult to terminate their relationship. Social workers, with their training and skill in the process of service termination, are particularly qualified to facilitate the timely termination of hospice services to the family.

Sometimes, however, hospice services provided to a patient in one type of setting may need to be terminated when the patient is transferred to another setting. For example, a hospitalized patient in an inpatient hospice unit may be released to home hospice care; a home hospice patient may decide to enter a freestanding hospice; or a patient who has been receiving noncertified home hospice services on an out-of-pocket basis may decide to enter a nursing home and apply for hospice services there through a Medicaid-certified hospice agency to become eligible for Medicaid coverage. In such situations, there may be financial, psychological, informational, or practical barriers to resolve.

Client Health Problems and Their Effects

Diagnoses. According to the National Association for Home Care (1996), in 1994, 58.7 percent of hospice patients had a primary diagnosis of "neoplasms" when admitted to hospice care; an additional 12.8 percent had a primary diagnosis of circulatory system disease; 6.7 percent had a disease of the nervous system or a sense organ; 6.6 percent had a respiratory system health problem; 3.1 percent had an infectious or parasitic disease; and the remaining 12 percent were distributed among a variety of other health disorders.

Physical suffering. People who have terminal health conditions often experience a variety of associated physical discomforts, such as pain, breathing difficulty, physical weakness, eating and sleeping problems, digestion and excretion problems, and sometimes sensory impairment, paralysis, skin problems, or swallowing difficulty (Fish, 1994; Germain, 1984:183). Effective pain control is central to hospice care and is a highly technical subject (Doyle, 1994). According to Buckingham (1996), physician home visits are not currently covered by Medicare, Medicaid, or private insurance (64), and many physicians write *PRN*, or "as needed," orders for pain medication. This can result in ineffective pain control because hospice staff wait until the patient is having pain before administering medication to relieve it (69).

Emotional and spiritual distress. With or without such physical discomfort and functional impairments, hospice patients also often experience considerable emotional distress—such as fear of dying, losing control, being alone, socially rejected, and feeling helpless, as well as apprehensions regarding "unfinished business," regrets about the past, or the distress of having family members burdened because of them (Germain, 1984:184; Allison, Gripton, and Rodway, 1990:207).

Family Member Problems and Needs

Family members are regarded as part of the client system, with their own problems and needs, such as the following:

- Lack of respite (mental and physical)
- Mental and physical exhaustion
- Social isolation or loss of external social life
- Financial needs
- Loss of employment income due to caregiving
- Anticipatory grief
- Unresolved conflicted relationships with the patient
- Generalized feelings of "stress" from all of these, in addition to the helpless sense that the patient cannot be saved
- Grief after the patient dies

As Fish (1994) wrote:

> It is in these areas of psychosocial and emotional problems that social workers can have an impact on the lives of patients and families. (408)

Social Worker Functions and Interventions

Objectives of Hospice Care

One approach to conceptualizing social worker functions and interventions is to think about the objectives of hospice care as follows:

- Relief of suffering
- Preservation of important relationships
- Facilitation of anticipatory grief
- Resolution of residual conflicts
- Supporting the clients' sense of integrity and control over decisions of importance to them (Weisman, 1972, cited in Moore, 1984:269)

Hospice Social Worker Functions

Thus, the broad function of social work in hospice care is to maximize the adjustment of hospice patients and their families to the challenges they face (Richman, 1995:1351).

Hospice Social Worker Roles

This broad function is performed through roles that Richman (1995) describes as broker, liaison, administrator, counselor, educator, lobbyist, and program planner, that is:

1. providing information and financial assistance [broker],
2. interfacing with the community [liaison],
3. administering and managing [hospice] agencies [administrator],
4. doing clinical work with individuals and families [counselor], and
5. promoting the acceptance of hospice philosophy and care by patients, the health care system, and society as a whole [educator, program planner, lobbyist]. (1361)

Fish (1994:410) cites some main tasks of social workers in hospice care as named by Pilsecker (1979):

1. Help patients and families to
   a. get in touch with their feelings and to understand their options;
   b. develop or maintain meaningful communication; and
   c. locate and use needed community resources.

2. Help other involved health professionals to
   a. get in touch with and acknowledge their own feelings;
   b. understand and respect patient and family needs; and
   c. meet patient and family needs in a sensitive manner.

Hospice Social Worker Roles in an Acute Hospital Setting

Stark and Johnson (1983) have explored social worker roles with terminally ill patients, families, staff, and students in an oncology unit of an acute care hospital, which may be summarized as follows:

1. Roles with patients and families:
   - Counseling
   - Advocacy
   - Liaison to community resources
   - Informant to facilitate informed decisions
   - Mediating as needed between patient, family, and staff
2. Roles with staff and students:
   - Collaboration, coordination, facilitation of team effort
   - Educating new staff/students about hospice concepts
   - Educating new staff/students about relevant community resources
   - Supportive counseling as needed

Effects of a hospice experience on acute care staff. Stark and Johnson (1983) report a number of *serendipitous effects* of their efforts to develop a hospice service within the teaching hospital oncology service where they were employed:

1. Increased attention to symptom control by all disciplines in the hospital as they developed understanding of the hospice philosophy
2. Increased comfort in shifting goals from curing to caring
3. More awareness of the need for patient and family to have options clearly presented, time allowed for them to process the information, and support and assistance if needed in making decisions
4. Increased appreciation of the advantages to staff of being involved in work with a variety of patients at all stages of dis-

ease, allowing them the feeling of having fulfilled a commitment to help the person live until he or she dies, and providing
an opportunity to work with the person's family
5. A growing awareness of the advantage of having the experience of working with dying patients and their families, available to students of all disciplines, an experience they can take
with them into their professional lives (68)

Hospice Social Worker Roles
in a Nursing Home Setting

Amar (1994) explored the difference between social work with
hospice patients and families in a nursing home setting compared
with that in a home care setting. Amar found nursing home patients
to be older and frailer, with more chronic health problems and
poorer mental health status, and thus less amenable to "talk therapies" (18-19); also, with less family support available, patients
were more vulnerable to the organizational environment, culture,
and competence of the nursing home and its staff. Thus, person-in-
environment "fit" between nursing home patient and nursing home
environment becomes crucial to effective social work with hospice
patients in such a setting.

Amar (1994) argues that the hospice social worker attending
nursing home patients has entered a more complex organizational
situation. The hospice program, affiliated with an outside organization, the patient and his or her family, and the nursing home organization—all have things the others want, and the social worker
needs to take care to mediate fairly between them. The hospice and
nursing home organizations have economic interests at stake. Hospice social work in a nursing home calls for more group work,
negotiation, education, and advocacy, and the focus of attention is
expanded from patient and family to include also nursing home and
hospice staff (Amar, 1994:22).

Psychosocial Assessment in Hospice Social Work

Presumably, most hospice social workers would agree with Quig
(1989:22-23), who saw that the essence of social work in hospice

care ought to revolve around *psychosocial assessment* and *support-ive counseling* with the patient and family—by working with pa-tients and families and their interactions, using a systems or ecolog-ical perspective.

Fish (1994) places fundamental importance on skilled psycho-social assessment by the social worker as the key to appropriate hospice team services to the patient and family:

> Assessing for strengths and weaknesses, coping strategies and defenses, communication patterns, availability of social sup-port beyond the nuclear and extended families, the need for legal or financial assistance and interpreting these issues to other team members helps the entire team to better understand the overall situation and to plan care within the appropriate framework. (408)

Lusk (1983) has presented a psychosocial history outline adapted to social work in hospice care (see Table 7.1). However, readers who wish to use this psychosocial assessment tool are urged to read Lusk's (1983) article, in which he elaborates a rationale for each part of the outline in a way that will facilitate and maximize the utility of the outline as a social work tool. Lusk (1983) reminds us:

> A psychosocial evaluation of a patient is an important first step in the provision of care to hospice patients and their families. It serves as a guide for intervention . . . hospice recognizes the uniqueness of each individual as he or she confronts life's final challenge. An adequate psychosocial evaluation brings that uniqueness into focus. (217)

Another potential function of such a psychosocial history is that it can serve as a *life review* or *oral history* for the patient and be instrumental in helping elderly people, especially, to achieve a sense of ego integrity. However, an interesting question for further research is how such a life review affects a terminally ill person who is not expected to reach "old age."

The Issue of a Unique Function for Hospice Social Work

According to McDonald (1991:274-275), a wide variety of roles and functions and activities have been allocated to hospice social

TABLE 7.1. Psychosocial Assessment of the Hospice Care Client

I. Basic Information (name, marital status, diagnosis, etc.)
II. Social History

  A. Developmental History
    1. Family system background
    2. Educational and occupational history
    3. Significant losses and crises
    4. Ethnic and cultural considerations

  B. Current Family System
    1. Size and structure
    2. Stability
    3. Caregivers and supporters
    4. Possible problem areas

III. Physical Resources

  A. Source and adequacy of income
  B. Medical insurance
  C. Need for services or referrals
    1. Financial services
    2. Medical equipment
    3. Social services
  D. Postmortem arrangements

IV. Psychosocial Functioning

  A. Mental Status
    1. Level of consciousness
    2. Orientation
    3. Memory and cognitive functions
    4. Appearance and expression
    5. Mood and affect
    6. Appropriateness of behavior

  B. Patient's Reaction to Illness
    1. Stage of grief
    2. Defense mechanisms
    3. Reactions to increased dependence

  C. Family's Reaction to Illness
    1. Stages of grief
    2. Defense mechanisms
    3. Reactions to patient's increased dependence
    4. Relationship between primary caregiver and patient

  D. Role impairment
    1. Patient's role in family
    2. Roles affected by illness
    3. Responsibilities reallocated to others

Source: Lusk, Mark (1983). The psychosocial evaluation of the hospice patient. *Health and Social Work,* 8: 211.

workers in the social work literature. These include referral, broker-age, generic problem-solving services, supportive and bereavement counseling, psychosocial assessment, case management, client advocacy, staff training and support, crisis intervention, hospice legislation reform, research, and community education.

Potential Areas for Development of Hospice Social Worker Function

However, what little research has been done on what social workers actually do in hospice programs suggests a general lack of unique role or function and considerable role overlap with other disciplines, especially nursing (McDonald, 1991:275). McDonald reports that his own observations from interactions with social workers and other hospice workers at meetings of the New York State Hospice Association concur with the findings of the Kulys and Davis study in 1986: that "non-social workers regularly provide psychosocial care in hospice and that financial and civil-legal assistance are the only functions that nurses and other team members unambiguously attribute to hospice social work" (McDonald, 1991:276).

Research, political activism, and community organization. Still, McDonald argues that hospice social workers may need to think more about other hospice needs, such as research, political activism, and community organization (1991:279), since a glance at the demographics of hospice clients reveals underrepresentation of people of color, the poor, and the uninsured. Also, funding is often inadequate to provide all the services needed by the patient and family; in addition to which, hospice programs have tended toward increased client load and paperwork, while sacrificing quality of patient and family services.

Psychosocial pain control techniques. Rodway and Blythe (1994) report from the findings of a study they conducted in 1988 that few hospice social workers were engaged in such potentially useful pain control interventions as relaxation therapy, hypnosis, or meditation (424).

Facilitating a pleasant physical environment. Another area of potential development for social work includes attending to the physical environment of the patient, such as facilitating the provision of a room that is pleasantly decorated and comfortable to the patient.

Improving the adequacy of bereavement and other psychosocial services. Rodway and Blythe (1994) also express concern that hospice programs tend to give considerable "lip service" to the value of bereavement counseling and psychosocial services to patient and family, but in practice often fail to demonstrate understanding of the need for organized, consistent, psychosocial services provided by qualified professionals (426). According to Buckingham (1996), hospice programs generally only provide bereavement services to families at 90 and 180 days after the death, with some variation across programs (74).

Bereavement service to grieving children. It is important to remember that oftentimes those grieving the loss of the relative are children. Sontag, Nadig, and Henry (1994) have reported a very useful description of imaginative ways to help children to express and work through their grief. The therapeutic medium was group work, and the social worker employed techniques such as helping the children (1) share with the group their stories of the person who died and the circumstances of the death; (2) share a photograph and biography of the deceased with the group; (3) express their feelings about their loss at a special time set aside in the group; (4) learn relaxation and physical health exercises; and (5) talk about their conceptions of death and afterlife. Each child also compiles a "memory book" of the deceased to keep, and the social worker helps the parents individually with their own grief and with knowing how to help their children with theirs.

Outreach to grieving others. Social workers need to remember that it is not only children who have difficulty dealing with death and their feelings of grief; we all do, to varying degrees. Certainly men, in particular, tend to have more difficulty expressing their feelings and thus are likely to be burdened with unresolved grief for a longer time.

Perhaps hospice organizations someday will assume responsibility for recruiting volunteers to read daily the obituary page of the local newspapers and reach out to every family who has had a recent death among them—to explore how they are doing and inform them of local resources for assistance, such as grief support groups. This would likely serve also as a form of "primary prevention" of health problems and premature death of the bereaved.

KNOWLEDGE REQUIREMENTS

In addition to generic social work knowledge, hospice social workers need to have hospice-specific knowledge concerning (1) the client population and client problem(s), (2) the organizational setting, (3) the community and its resources, (4) intervention modalities, and (5) needed research, evaluation, and documentation.

The Client Population

Health Condition

Perhaps the one common denominator within the hospice patient population is that all patients are facing fairly imminent death, usually estimated as within six months. For this reason, hospice social workers need to come to terms with their own feelings and attitudes toward death before they can hope to help others with their grief and bereavement (Moore, 1984). In this instance, knowledge cannot be reduced to familiarity with facts and theories, but must include some experiences that help to develop empathy. Moore reported a sensitivity training program for hospice social workers that involved the following kinds of exercises:

1. Complete a multiple choice questionnaire concerning your past experiences, present beliefs, and personal perceptions relating to death.
2. Write down what you would want to accomplish if you had ten years to live. Then repeat the task for the different intervals of five years, one year, one month, and, finally, one week.
3. Make up your own obituary as it would be written today, and as it would be written in your old age.
4. Imagine yourself arriving at a cemetery, spotting your own tombstone, and seeing what was written on the stone in memoriam.

5. Write a letter to someone deceased, addressing "unfinished business" and unresolved feelings, sign it and share it with someone else if you wish.
6. Imagine you had received a telegram informing you of the imminent death (within minutes) of a significant other. You had five minutes to say your last words to that person. (Moore, 1984:270)

Moore (1984:271) also describes a series of concluding exercises that help to counteract the participants' sense of emotional exhaustion. Moore implies that such exercises as previously described can be quite traumatic to persons with compromised coping capacity and are not to be engaged in indiscriminately.

To work effectively in a hospice setting, the social worker must understand who the patients are and the significance of their characteristics, both healthwise and demographic. Thus, it is important to understand how, for example, young women with terminal breast cancer differ from children with terminal leukemia, or from young gay men with AIDS, or from old people with congestive heart failure. In addition to understanding the nature and implications of patients' particular health conditions, one also needs to have a sense of the demographic characteristics of the hospice population, including ethnicity, age, sex, and marital status, and how these characteristics are similar or different from the general population.

Ethnicity. In 1994, 80.8 percent of hospice patients were white, 7.2 percent were black, and the other 12 percent were of unknown ethnic identity. This suggests that whites are overrepresented in hospice care, as only about 75 percent of the general population was classed as white at that time. Conversely, since about 12 percent of the general population was black, the 7.2 percent figure suggests that blacks are underrepresented in formal hospice care (U.S. Government Printing Office, 1995:134).

Age. Furthermore, in 1994, 69.1 percent of hospice patients were age sixty-five and older, and within this age group, the largest percentage were age eighty-five and older—reflecting the correlation between increasing age and increasing death rates. Although the majority of hospice patients are elderly, 9.0 percent of hospice patients are under age forty-five (U.S. Government Printing Office, 1995:134).

Sex. Also in 1994, somewhat more hospice patients were female than male, that is, 55.3 percent female and 44.7 percent male (U.S. Government Printing Office, 1995:134).

Marital status. Finally, in 1994, nearly 50 percent of hospice patients were married (48.4 percent), 30.6 percent widowed, 6 percent divorced or separated, 11.4 percent never married, and the remaining 3.7 were of unknown marital status (U.S. Government Printing Office, 1995:134).

The Organizational Setting

As indicated earlier, it is important to understand the nature of the hospice organization—whether affiliated with a hospital, home care agency, nursing home, hospice inpatient facility, or a freestanding organization. It is also important to know how it may differ from other hospice organizations, due to affiliation with some religious group, the personality of the current director, the policy of its funding sources, or other influence such as community or regional attitudes and values.

It is necessary to realize that hospice philosophy and values tend to represent an alternative paradigm to the rest of the health care system, in that the focus is on process more than product, on a qualitative service rather than a quantitative outcome. According to Gummer (1988), hospice programs are based on the alternative paradigm that "function follows form," and so they emphasize three functions of organizational form: (1) the primacy of process over product, (2) power equalization with participatory decision-making, and (3) small size to encourage intimacy.

In short, what matters most is the quality of the interaction of hospice workers with patients and families, the empowerment of patients and families through influencing decision making, and the maintenance of relationships among them all that are characterized by mutual support and affection. Hospice objectives are achieved as a result of these structural patterns.

The Community and Its Resources

The hospice social worker needs to know what policies and programs are available to assist hospice clients. Most hospice patients are in home care situations, where they not only often need Medicare or Medicaid financing to pay for their care but also such resources as home-delivered meals, tool and equipment rentals, support groups for family caregivers, and visits from friends and neighbors.

The culture of a community can impact on attitudes and readiness to help victims of certain types of problems. For example, some communities may be ignorant and fearful or superstitious about certain health conditions, such as cancer or AIDS.

The more rural the community, the less specialized or "high tech" the resources it is likely to have. In such areas, alternative resources often need to be explored.

Intervention Modalities

The hospice social worker requires a repertoire of effective interventions to address particular needs of clients. The psychosocial assessment of the patient and family determines which approaches are selected. For example, choice of intervention depends on the extent to which they need information and referral, pain control, skill development, supportive counseling, behavioral change, cognitive change, improved intrafamily communication and understanding, environmental modification, social support networking, empowerment and development of coping skills, or advocacy. Hospice social worker functions and interventions were discussed earlier in this chapter under Social Worker Functions and Interventions.

Needed Research, Evaluation, and Documentation

Dush (1988a, 1988b) points out that although nurses and other hospice care workers have tended to assume social worker responsibilities in the area of psychosocial assessment and treatment, little research has been done to develop knowledge about which particular intervention modalities work best with particular types of clients or client problems.

What was said about home health care research and evaluation applies to social work in hospice care as well (see Chapter 5), and, as always, the social worker needs to know the documentation requirements of the service provider and funding source and take care to accurately and completely comply with these requirements to ensure continued support for social work services. In the past, errors in documentation have sometimes resulted in reimbursement losses and reductions in use of that discipline by the service provider.

VALUES AND ETHICS CONSIDERATIONS

The values and ethics of the social work profession are remarkably compatible with those of hospice care. Above all, anyone working with a hospice program must be able to value every human individual, the principle of client confidentiality, human diversity, social justice and commitment to serve vulnerable populations, and client self-determination.

Stark and Johnson (1983) described the efforts of the teaching hospital in which they worked as social workers to incorporate a hospice service within the oncology inpatient service. They noted some ethical issues that were raised:

- What constitutes ordinary versus extraordinary means?
- How should the social worker be involved in this decision?
- To whom should the social worker be responsible when there is an irreconcilable conflict concerning patient care decisions between patient and family or between patient/family and physicians? (68-69)

Since most hospice care is provided in the home, much of what was said about values and ethics in home health care applies as well to hospice care (see Chapter 5). In addition, some of the more obvious social worker values and ethics challenges to which hospice social work is most vulnerable include the following hypothetical examples:

- The social worker perceives an important unmet need of the patient and/or family that the hospice organization and/or funding source is unwilling or unable to meet.

- The patient or family tells the social worker something in confidence that other team members ought to know.
- The social worker learns that the hospice agency is charging for services that were not provided.
- The social worker finds that the hospice agency is violating some rule or failing to meet some standard of the funding or certifying organization.
- The social worker is offered an exciting employment opportunity elsewhere, but one or more hospice patients and their families have grown exceedingly dependent on the social worker for understanding and emotional support and indicate that they "couldn't make it" if the social worker left.

SKILL REQUIREMENTS

Professional skill is the ability to perform well whatever activity is involved in one's work and must reflect the integration of relevant knowledge as well as values and ethics. Such skill is used while interacting with a complex set of variable conditions; therefore, true professional skill is conscious, purposeful, disciplined, and responsible.

It is not enough to "care about" people; one also needs to know how to help them and how to "take care" of them. Unfortunately, failure to understand this results in much wasted effort, as well as actual harm, by well-meaning but unqualified helpers in the name of "caring."

COMMENTARY

Hospice social work is not for every social worker or other health professional. However, anecdotal reports from people who do hospice work often claim that it is the most rewarding experience of their lives, even if they were not immediately attracted to it. Thus, the reader is urged not to rule it out without a closer look through a practicum experience.

CROSS-CULTURAL RESOURCES

Ford, Gillian (1993). Hospice in England—A palliative care system: The Marie Curie model. *The American Journal of Hospice and Palliative Care,* (July/August): 27-29.

Johanson, Gary A. (1993). Palliative care in Argentina: A gringo's perspective. *The American Journal of Hospice and Palliative Care,* (July/August): 11-12.

Kerr, Derek (1993). Lin zhong guan huai: Terminal care in China. *The American Journal of Hospice and Palliative Care,* (July/August): 18-26.

Parry, Joan K. and Ryan, Angela Shen (Eds.) (1995). *A cross-cultural look at death, dying, and religion.* Chicago: Nelson-Hall.

Rosner, Fred (1993). Hospice, medical ethics, and Jewish customs. *The American Journal of Hospice and Palliative Care,* (July/August): 6-10.

Storey, Porter (1993). Hospice settings around the world. *The American Journal of Hospice and Palliative Care,* (July/August): 4-5.

Suzuki, Shizue, Kirsschling, Jane Marie, and Inoue, Iku (1993). Hospice care in Japan. *The American Journal of Hospice and Palliative Care,* (July/August): 35-40.

Zylicz, Zbigniew (1993). Hospice in Holland: The story behind the blank spot. *The American Journal of Hospice and Palliative Care,* (July/August): 30-34.

SECTION III:
HEALTH SERVICE DELIVERY
AND FINANCING

Chapter 8

U.S. Health Care System Strengths and Problems

DESCRIPTION AND ASSESSMENT OF THE SYSTEM

Economic Access to Health Services

The U.S. "nonsystem" of economic access to health care services represents a "mixed model" with the following features: (1) *Medicare*, which amounts to national health insurance for selected groups (elderly and disabled who are eligible for Social Security, as well as persons who are medically dependent upon expensive renal dialysis treatments for survival as a result of end-stage renal disease), financed from employee payroll taxes; (2) *Medicaid*, a public assistance program financed from state and federal general revenues for persons who qualify for subsistence income assistance from government programs, in addition to low-income pregnant women and children, with types of coverage and benefit levels varying across state programs; and (3) *private health insurance* coverage for most employed persons, financed, in full or in part, by their employers.

The Uninsured Population

Unfortunately, these three basic sources of health insurance coverage do not fit together in such a way that all Americans are included; rather, they leave gaps in the "patchwork" that cause a substantial portion of the population to go without any coverage. In 1995, 15.4 percent of the U.S. population, or about forty million persons, were without any health insurance—Medicaid, Medicare, or private health insurance (U.S. Government Printing Office, 1997b:120).

Recent increase in uninsured. The size of the uninsured population has increased in recent years. The percentage of Americans
without health insurance coverage increased from 12.9 percent in
1987 to 15.4 percent in 1995 (U.S. Government Printing Office,
1997b:120).

Geographical variation. The size of the uninsured population
varies across states within the United States. Depending on the
state, in 1995, the uninsured population percentage ranged from a
low of 7.3 percent in Wisconsin to a high of 25.6 percent in New
Mexico (U.S. Government Printing Office, 1997b:120).

Ethnic variation. As is the case with most advantages in the United
States, racial and ethnic minority group members tend to fair worse
than the white majority. In the United States, in 1995, 14.2 percent of
whites, 21 percent of blacks, and 33.3 percent of Hispanics had no
health insurance (U.S. Government Printing Office, 1997b:120).

Age variation. Across age groups, the elderly are most advantaged
in terms of health insurance coverage; less than 1 percent (0.9 percent)
of persons age sixty-five and over were without health insurance in
1995, while 28.2 percent of young adults ages eighteen to twenty-four,
22.9 percent of young adults ages twenty-five to thirty-four, and
13.8 percent of children under age eighteen had no health coverage
(U.S. Government Printing Office, 1997b:120).

Employment status. According to Billings (1999), "the profile of
the typical uninsured person might be a young adult in a low-wage
job working for a small employer in the retail/service sector of the
economy . . . more than half of the uninsured earn less than 10,000
per year, and 85 percent earn less than $20,000" (406).

The Underinsured Population

In addition to the uninsured population, a large segment of the
U.S. population has only partial health insurance coverage, requiring
out-of-pocket contributions in the form of deductibles, coinsurance,
and simply uncovered services. In 1995, Americans' out-of-pocket
expenses were 3.3 percent of total costs of hospital care, 36.7 percent of nursing home care costs, 18.3 percent of total physicians'
services, and 42.4 percent of all other *personal health care expenditures*—or about 20.8 percent of all personal health care expenditures

of $878 billion, 800 million (U.S. Government Printing Office, 1997a:260). Altogether, in 1994, Americans expended out-of-pocket payments totaling $182 billion, 563 million, or about 18.5 percent of all *national health expenditures* of $988 billion, 489 million (U.S. Government Printing Office, 1997b:112). Note that national health expenditures includes not only personal health care expenditures (such as health services and supplies and insurance premiums) but also such things as medical research and medical facilities construction.

The Original Intent and Current Outcomes of the Medicare and Medicaid Programs

Reflecting perhaps the disadvantages of a "residual" approach to social welfare policy and programs, neither Medicare nor Medicaid have developed as their authors intended. In an interesting piece about the history of Medicare (Title XVIII of the Social Security Act), passed by Congress in 1965, Robert M. Ball (1996), consultant on Social Security, who was instrumental in getting the Medicare policy enacted, and who is a past commissioner of Social Security and a current member of the Social Security Advisory Council, laid out the history of efforts to pass national health insurance legislation in the United States. He explained that he and all the others who developed and fought for the passage of Medicare saw it as a "last ditch" effort to obtain national health insurance for all Americans. It was never intended to be permanently limited to health insurance for the elderly only. Instead, targeting the elderly was a planned political strategy based on the following assumptions: the public would be most sympathetic to this group; the American Medical Association (AMA) would have a harder time opposing a program to help older people; and hospitals would tend to favor having a means for being reimbursed for care of older patients, who in the past were often unable to pay their hospital bills because they were retired and without employer-provided private health insurance.

On the other hand, Medicaid (Title XIX of the Social Security Act), also passed in 1965, was originally intended to provide health insurance for public assistance recipients, such as AFDC (Aid to Families with Dependent Children) families (Lyons, Rowland, and

Hanson, 1996). However, due to the long-term care limitations of Medicare coverage for the elderly and the lack of other insurance coverage for many indigent and disabled persons, by 1993 only 27 percent of Medicaid funds were used for health care for welfare recipients, while 28 percent of Medicaid spending paid for nursing home and home care for the elderly (most of which is not covered under Medicare), 31 percent for health care for disabled people, and the other 14 percent went to DPS (disproportionate share) hospitals—that is, hospitals providing extensive health care services to the poor and uninsured (Lyons, Rowland, and Hanson, 1996).

Although Medicaid was originally intended to provide economic access to health care for the poor population, as of 1994, only 46 percent of the U.S. population with income below the government "poverty line" was covered by Medicaid (Karger and Stoesz, 1998).

Types of Health Service Organizations

A "mixed model" form also characterizes the health services themselves, in that the hospitals, nursing homes, home care agencies, outpatient clinics, and other organizational settings of such services are sometimes public tax-supported ones, sometimes private non-profit, and sometimes private for-profit ones. The current trend is toward domination by the for-profit sector, except for hospitals and hospice organizations, where, despite an increase in for-profit hospital and hospice organizations, the nonprofit sector continues to predominate. As of 1996, only about 20.7 percent of U.S. hospitals were operated for profit (Woolhandler and Himmelstein, 1997:770), and in 1994, only 7.3 percent of hospice organizations were proprietary ones (U.S. Government Printing Office, 1995:135).

Health Service Payer Trends

However, although a growing percentage of organizations providing health services are proprietary/for-profit ones, an increasing percentage of health care costs, about 44 percent, are covered through public tax-supported programs, such as Medicare, Medicaid, and the VA; the remaining 56 percent of health care costs through private programs are largely (84 percent) paid for by employers (Friedland, 1996). The share of hospital care paid by government health insurance and other government health programs increased from 42.5 percent in 1960 to 61.2 percent in 1995; for nursing home care, it rose from 15.7 percent in 1960 to 58.1 percent in 1995; for physicians' services, it rose from 7.1 percent in 1960 to 31.7 percent in 1995; and for all other personal health care, it increased from 8.1 percent in 1960 to 27.5 percent in 1995 (U.S. Government Printing Office, 1997a:260).

The Quality of Health Care

If one can afford it, almost any desired health care service or procedure is available in America, and often at a very high quality—including not only routine interventions but also cosmetic surgeries, organ transplants, and joint replacements. Overall, most Americans are very satisfied with the health care services they receive (Zis, Jacobs, and Shapiro, 1996), and professional health care providers, such as physicians, nurses, and allied health care professionals (e.g., social workers, physical therapists, occupational therapists, and speech therapists) are generally well trained, with high legal and professional practice standards.

It is common to hear Americans exclaim that "the United States has the best health care in the world; that's why people who can afford to come here from all over the world for health services they can't get in their own countries!" or "If the Canadian health care system is so great, why do so many Canadians come to the United States for services they can't get in their own country?" (The second comment is generally made in reference to some Canadians who pay for elective, nonurgent procedures in the United States rather than waiting for them to be scheduled and covered by National Health Insurance in Canada.)

What American comments are responding to, apparently, is what has been coined "the proliferation of technology" in U.S. health care. Newhouse (1996), Director of the Division of Health Policy Research and Education at Harvard University, has asserted that the major cause of increased health care costs probably is the tremendous increase in medical "capability," that is, technology.

Yet, Harry E. Simmons (1996), President of the National Leadership Coalition of Health Care, has said that "the three serious and interrelated problems facing our health care system . . . are rising costs, decreasing coverage, and problems in quality" (57). Simmons attributes the fact that "our per capita health care costs are almost double those of other developed nations" (57) to excessive use of technology, in that we tend to use it even when the resultant benefits are not established. In fact, many medical and surgical interventions employed by U.S. physicians are not well grounded in outcomes research; both the quantity of medical care and the types of interventions vary widely across geographical regions, with a lack of evidence regarding variance in outcomes (Simmons, 1996; Kane, 1995:13, 15).

All this reflects a greater lack of scientific knowledge in medicine than we tend to assume (Simmons, 1996). In addition, technology is sometimes knowingly misused, for example, due to pressure from patients to give antibiotics for a cold, pressure from hospitals to use expensive equipment, such as an MRI (magnetic resonance imaging) to help pay for it, or pressure from patients or families, or physicians' own internal pressure, to "do something," even when curative interventions for the problem are not known.

Furthermore, the error rate in medical interventions may well exceed the annual rate of fatal auto accidents, indicating a serious lack of quality control and challenging the use of patient satisfaction surveys as a measure of the quality of our health care system (Simmons, 1996). In short, improvement in the quality of health care through better knowledge of comparative outcomes of interventions, fewer medical errors, and proper use of interventions could significantly reduce health care costs (Simmons, 1996).

Health Care Costs

Interestingly, Medicare recipients have been found to be more satisfied with their health insurance plan than employed people, Medicaid recipients, or unemployed people, and Medicare has lower administrative costs than private health insurance programs (Lave, 1996). According to Lave (1996), the causes of the high costs of clinical services covered by Medicare include a combination of technology changes, the focus of Medicare coverage on acute care rather than both preventive and long-term supportive care services, as well as the general tendency to try to control costs through price controls, deductibles, and coinsurance rather than by changing utilization incentives.

Reviewing trends in health care reforms worldwide, all of which appear directed at controlling health care costs, Kirkman-Liff (1996) lists the common features of these directions as follows:

1. Use of a national global health care budget to achieve cost control
2. Shifting management responsibility from government to private/quasi-private institutions
3. Capitation paid to primary group-medical practices
4. Use of primary care physicians as "gatekeepers" to the rest of the health care system
5. Encouragement of medical practice in group or health center settings
6. Financial incentives to physicians to focus on health maintenance
7. Prospective payments to hospitals (e.g., DRGs), or risk-based contracts with hospitals to cover a population, often paid by primary care physician groups (e.g., HMOs) from capitated budgets
8. Integration of specialists with hospitals
9. Consumer choice of provider-integrated networks (managed care organizations) under contract with a primary care physician group budget-holder or health insurer budget-holder
10. A guaranteed minimal set of services assured to all citizens
11. Individual freedom to purchase supplemental health service insurance (69)

One of the issues in health care is whether nonprofit or for-profit health care organizations are better. One side of this issue concerns the quality of care, while the other side of the coin is relative cost/benefit.

Two relevant tendencies in public opinion in America today include (1) confusing a "free market" economic system with freedom and democracy in the political system and (2) an assumption that "market principles" will make health or social welfare programs more efficient for the same reasons they tend to produce efficiency in other business and industrial operations.

However, some evidence is beginning to emerge that challenges these assumptions. For example, a large study (Woolhandler and Himmelstein, 1997) was recently reported that compared the costs during 1994, according to Medicare reports submitted by hospitals, of the three organizational types of hospitals. The study found that the for-profit hospitals cost significantly more than nonprofit or public hospitals in terms of (1) the average percentage of the hospital's budget devoted to administration, (2) the average cost per inpatient day, and (3) the average cost per discharge/inpatient stay. On the other hand, for-profit hospitals also had lower costs/overhead for employee wages, salaries, and benefits (raising issues of the quality of services). Administrative costs of for-profit psychiatric and rehabilitation hospitals, which are exempt from DRGs, were found to be especially higher. Woolhandler and Himmelstein (1997) noted:

> Even before these recent rises in expenditure for administration, the U.S. General Accounting Office calculated that the administrative savings that would result from a shift to national health insurance would fully fund universal coverage. (774) (Woolhandler, Steffie and Himmelstein, David U. 1997. Costs of care and administration at for-profit and other hospitals in the United States. *New England Journal of Medicine,* 336[11]:769-799. Copyright © 1997 Massachusetts Medical Society. All rights reserved.)

Given this, it is amazing to hear leaders of health care professions or organizations publicly assert that, in spite of rising health care costs in the United States, the solution is not to shift to a system of national health insurance, such as in Canada, because it would only increase costs further.

Curiously, Canadians utilize more physician and hospital services than Americans do, and administrative costs in the Canadian health care system are significantly less than those in the United States (Rachlis, 1997:144, 146). Surely, it is not coincidental that the United States is the only industrialized nation in the world, besides South Africa, without a national system for ensuring universal economic access to basic health care, yet the United States also spends considerably more, both per capita and in terms of GDP, on health care than any of these other industrialized societies, all of which have national health insurance, a national health service, or other system of universal economic access to basic health care.

The U.S. Government Printing Office (1997b:835) provides some comparative data on health expenditures in the United States and twenty-eight other industrial nations, according to both percentage of GDP as well as per capita. The data show that in 1995, the U.S. expended 14.2 percent of its GDP on health care, compared with Germany, the next highest at 10.4 percent, while twenty of the twenty-eight countries spent less than 9 percent.

In addition, the United States spent $3,701 per capita for health care during 1995, and Switzerland was the next highest in terms of per capita health care costs that year, at $2,412. Canada, whose health care system Americans often claim they could not afford, expended $2,049 per capita for health care in 1995, a mere 55 percent of U.S. expenditures for health care, while both Sweden and Denmark, which are known for their very generous universal health and welfare systems, each expended a little over $1,300 per capita in 1995—less than 40 percent of U.S. health care costs (see Table 8.1).

Cost-Benefit Issues

Americans like to assert that the United States has the best health care system in the world—in spite of the fact that the United States ranks lower than many other nations in terms of basic indicators of population health status, such as life expectancy and infant mortality rate. In 1993, the infant mortality rate in the United States was 8.37 deaths of infants under one year out of every 1,000 live births; this is higher than twenty-four other industrial nations and almost twice as high as Japan's infant mortality rate of 4.35 the same year (U.S. Government Printing Office, 1997a:105); this was despite the fact that Japan spends less than one-half of what the United States does on health care per capita ($1,581 relative to $3,701) (U.S. Government Printing Office, 1997b:835). Yet Japan has the longest

TABLE 8.1. Health Care Expenditures, Life Expectancy, and Infant Mortality, United States and Selected Countries, 1993-1995

Country	1995 Expenditures %GDP**	$per capita**	1993 Life expectancy at birth (years)***	1993 Infant mortality per 1,000 births*
U.S.	14.2	3,701	72.2 m 78.8 f	8.37
Switzerland	9.8	2,412.(2)	75.0 m 81.7 f	5.55
Germany	10.4	2,134	72.8 m 79.3 f	5.84
Canada	9.6	2,049	74.9 m 81.4 f	6.30
France	9.8	1,956	73.8 m 82.3 f	6.82
Japan	7.2	1,581	76.5 m 83.1 f	4.35
Finland	7.7	1,373	72.1 m 79.6 f	4.40
Denmark	6.4	1,368	72.7 m 77.9 f	5.40
Sweden	7.2	1,360	75.5 m 80.8 f	4.84
United Kingdom	6.9	1,246	73.9 m 79.5 f	6.24

Sources:
* U.S. Government Printing Office (1997a). *Health, United States, 1996-1997.* Washington, DC: Author, 105.
** U.S. Government Printing Office (1997b). *Statistical Abstracts of the United States.* Washington, DC: Author, 835.
*** U.S. Government Printing Office (1997a). *Health, United States, 1996-1997.* Washington, DC: Author, 106.

life expectancy of any nation in the world, both at birth and at age sixty-five, for both males and females (U.S. Government Printing Office, 1997a:106). Table 8.1 illustrates some of this comparative data.

What is wrong with the U.S. health care system? In short, it is inefficient; we spend more on health care than any other country in the world, yet indicators of population health, such as infant mortality rate and life expectancy, show that we are well below many other nations in terms of the health status of our citizens. Perhaps it is time to consider the following proposal by Woolhandler and Himmelstein (1997):

> Since the gap between health care costs in the United States and those in the rest of the world is widening and the ranks of the uninsured and underinsured are swelling, perhaps it is time to ask whether our experiment with market medicine has failed. (774) (Woolhandler, Steffie and Himmelstein, David U. 1997. Costs of care and administration at for-profit and other hospitals in the United States. *New England Journal of Medicine*, 336[11]: 769-799. Copyright © 1997 Massachusetts Medical Society. All rights reserved.)

Distribution of U.S. health care expenditures. Table 8.2 shows that, in 1995, a total of $988.5 billion dollars was expended for health care. Over one-half (55.8 percent) of all U.S. health care expenditures went for only two categories: inpatient hospital services (35.4 percent) and physicians' services (20.4 percent). In contrast, only 3.2 percent of all health care expenditures went for government public health services. Presumably, most public health expenditures are for primary prevention, that is, efforts to prevent health problems from occurring, and early intervention, efforts to prevent problems from developing further.

Distribution of Medicare expenditures. Table 8.3 provides the distribution of health care expenditures through the Medicare program in 1995. The data show that $117 billion, 604 million was spent through Part A of Medicare and an additional $66 billion, 600 million through Part B of Medicare, for a total of $184 billion, 204 million combined, which is 18.6 percent of total national health care expenditures in 1995 in the United States.

Table 8.3 also illustrates that more than three-fourths (75.8 percent) of Medicare Part A expenditures in 1995 were for acute inpatient hospital care—the most expensive level of care—while the bulk (60.7 percent) of Medicare Part B expenditures were for out-patient physicians' services. *Long-term care*, or the combination of nursing home, home health, and hospice care, constituted only 23.3 percent of total Medicare expenditures.

TABLE 8.2. Distribution of U.S. National Health Expenditures, 1995, by Object, Percent, Billions of Dollars, and Rank Order

Ranking	Object	Percent	Billions of Dollars	Cumulative Percent
1	Hospital	35.4	350.1	35.4
2	Physician	20.4	201.6	55.8
3	Drugs and other medical nondurables	8.4	83.4	64.2
4	Nursing home	7.9	77.9	72.2
5	Other professional service	5.3	52.6	77.5
6	Insurance and administration	4.8	47.7	82.3
7	Dental	4.6	45.8	86.9
8	Government public health	3.2	31.4	90.1
9	Home health care	2.9	28.6	93.0
10	Other health services	2.5	25.0	95.5
11	Medical research	2.0	16.6	97.5
12	Medical facility construction	1.4	14.0	98.9
13	Vision products and other medical durables	1.4	13.8	100.3
Totals		100.2	988.5	

Sources: U.S. Government Printing Office (1997a). *Health, United States, 1996-1997.* Washington, DC: Author, 254; U.S. Government Printing Office (1997b). *Statistical Abstracts of the United States.* Washington, DC: Author, 112.

TABLE 8.3. Distribution of Medicare Expenditures, Part A and Part B, 1995, by Object, Amount, and Percent

Part A: Hospital Insurance:	Amount (Billions of Dollars)	Percent
Inpatient hospital	89.130	75.8
Skilled nursing facility	9.541	8.1
Home health agency	15.503	13.2
Hospice	2.002	1.7
Administrative expenses*	1.236	1.1
Total Part A	117.604	100.0
Part B: Supplementary Medical Insurance	Amount (Billions of Dollars)	Percent
Physician	40.457	60.7
Outpatient hospital	15.405	23.1
Home health agency	.182	0.3
Group practice prepayment	6.884	10.3
Independent laboratory	2.046	3.1
Administrative expenses*	1.627	2.4
Total Part B	66.600	100.0

Source: U.S. Government Printing Office (1997a). *Health, United States, 1996-1997.* Washington, DC: Author, 272.

* Includes costs of experiments, demonstration projects, and peer review activity.

Distribution of Medicaid expenditures. Table 8.4 indicates that over one-half (56.9 percent) of Medicaid expenditures in 1995 were for inpatient hospital or nursing home care, that is, institutional services, which are the first three categories listed. The total expended under the Medicaid program that year was $120 billion, 141 million, which was about 12.2 percent of total expenditures of $955.5 billion dollars for national health services that year. Note, too, that only one-half of 1 percent of Medicaid expenditures was used for family planning, an important aspect of preventive health care.

TABLE 8.4. Distribution of Medicaid Expenditures, 1995, by Object, Amount, and Percent

Object	Amount (Billions of Dollars)	Percent
Inpatient hospital: 　General hospital 　Mental hospital	26.331 2.511	22.0 2.1
Intermediate care facilities (mentally retarded)	10.383	8.6
Nursing facility services	29.052	24.2
Physicians	7.360	6.1
Dental	1.019	0.9
Other practitioner	0.966	0.8
Outpatient hospital	6.627	5.5
Clinic	4.280	3.6
Laboratory	1.180	1.0
Home health	9.406	8.0
Prescribed drugs	9.791	8.2
Family planning	0.514	0.5
Total	120.141	does not add to 100%

Source: U.S. Government Printing Office (1997a). *Health, United States, 1996-1997.* Washington, DC: Author, 118.

MANAGED CARE

The Background of Managed Care

Managed care has emerged in the United States as one category of effort to control health care costs, which continued to rise at an increasing rate until the *annual rate of increase* diminished to 11.6 percent for the period 1980 to 1985, down from 13.5 percent for the previous period of 1975 to 1980. The decreasing rate of increase apparently reflected the introduction in 1983 of the diagnosis-related group (DRG) system under Medicare, whereby hospitals no longer were reimbursed on a fee-for-service basis, but rather according to a system of standard payments based on the customary treatment and length of stay for that diagnosis. In addition, the decrease in the health care cost increase rate may have reflected the fact that health maintenance organizations more than doubled in number during that same period, 1980 to 1985 (U.S. Government Printing Office, 1997a:271). Amazingly, since 1985, the annual rate of increase in national health care expenditures has continued to decrease across subsequent periods and was last reported to be at an all-time low of only 5.5 percent for the one-year period of 1994 to 1995 (U.S. Government Printing Office, 1997a:254).

Still, the actual cost of national health care expenditures in the United States continued to increase, in spite of the reduction in the rate of increase. In 1985, national health care expenditures totaled $428.2 billion, but by 1995, they had more than doubled, reaching $988.5 billion (U.S. Government Printing Office, 1997a:254).

The Growth and Development of Managed Care

HMOs first emerged in the 1930s and 1940s, but since the 1970s, a new form of managed care has emerged, called "utilization review firms" or "managed care organizations." The idea behind this new form is that a third party other than the service provider or patient influences which kinds and amounts of service interventions will be approved for reimbursement. The motive is entirely cost control (Freeman and Trabin, 1994, cited in Manderscheid and Henderson, 1998:114). In fact, Munson (1997) has somewhat facetiously referred to managed care organizations as "managed cost organizations" (480).

HMOs had their roots in the nineteenth century in plantation owners, mining companies, and lumber firms providing health care services themselves (not health insurance) as a fringe benefit to attract and retain workers (Friedman, 1996, cited in Kovner, 1999:283). Similarly, the first true HMO was started in the 1930s when what has since become known as the Kaiser Permanente Health Plan was offered to recruit and retain workers to help build the Grand Coulee Dam in Washington and then to attract shipbuilding workers in Oakland, California, during World War II (Kovner, 1999:283).

During the administration of Richard Nixon (1969-1974), "The Health Maintenance Organization Act of 1973 (Public Law 93-222) stimulated a sluggish health maintenance industry that has since grown at an explosive rate" (Karger and Stoesz, 1998:187). The HMO Act of 1973 authorized federal aid to establish HMO facilities in many favorable marketing areas that, combined with the coexisting growth in the nursing home and hospital management industries, peaked investor interest. Within ten years of the HMO Act of 1973, sixty proprietary HMOs were operating (Karger and Stoesz, 1998:190).

Managed care organizations in the United States have grown from only 174 in 1976 to 628 such organizations in 1996, including 366 independent practice associations (IPAs), 122 group practice associations, and 140 mixed-model organizations (U.S. Government Printing Office, 1997a:271). The two periods of greatest increase in HMOs were between 1980 and 1985, when the number more than doubled, and between 1995 and 1996. The second growth spurt followed the political failure of the proposed Clinton Health Care Security Act of 1993.

As of 1996, nearly 20 percent (19.9 percent) of insured Americans were enrolled in managed care organizations; with the highest percentage (30.7 percent) in the west, 23.8 percent in the northeast, 16.2 percent in the midwest, and the lowest percentage (13.2 percent) in the southern part of the United States. This included 16.2 percent of Medicaid recipients and 7 percent of Medicare recipients (U.S. Government Printing Office, 1997a:271).

What Is "Managed Care"?

Managed care refers to a cluster of health service systems, including *health maintenance organizations* (HMOs), with the three main models of (1) group, (2) staff, (3) independent practice associations (IPAs), and (4) the newest form of HMO, provider service organizations (PSOs). Managed care includes also other forms (but not HMOs), such as preferred provider organizations (PPOs), and point-of-service plans (POSs).

I will try to clarify the distinguishing features of each variety of managed care model; however, it needs to be recognized that the literature is somewhat confusing because of the lack of consistent use of terms (especially the terms group model, staff model, and network model), as well as the variance in features, not only between models, but within models.

The Group Model (e.g., Kaiser Permanente)

According to Mechanic (1999):

> The traditional and most studied HMO type is the *group model* in which the insurance plan contracts with one or many large multispecialty groups on a capitated basis to provide services exclusively to its insured population. The professional group is responsible for its internal organization and processes and for distributing income within the group, but the insurance plan provides for hospitals or other needed physical facilities. These facilities may be directly owned by the plan, be available through contracts, or both. (154)

In the "group model," the provider organization, that is, the professional group, assumes the financial risk of providing services that cost more than the prepaid capitated sum.

The Staff Model (e.g., Group Health Cooperative of Puget Sound)

> Staff model HMOs are similar to group models in many ways, but physicians are typically salaried and not personally at risk, although there may be financial incentives to help shape their behavior. The insurance organization, however, is capitated and is at risk. Physicians tend to dislike staff models, which make physicians employees, and they commonly convert to group models over time. (Mechanic, 1999:154)

Independent Practice Association Model/Network Model

As of 1996, independent practice associations (IPAs) were the predominant model of managed care, constituting 58.3 percent of the 628 managed care organizations reported that year (U.S. Government Printing Office, 1997a:271). According to Mechanic (1999), the IPA model also is referred to as the "network model." The usual pattern is for the insuring organization to develop a network of physicians in solo practice, or group practice of the same specialty, who will serve the insurance enrollees. These are capitated insurance plans and the physicians also are often paid on a capitated basis. The physicians are not required to limit their services only to one HMO, but instead may participate in several and may also see fee-for-service patients. The advantage of the independent practice association, or network model, is that it provides more flexibility and autonomy to the physicians, and greater choice of physicians to patients. However, under the IPA model, the physicians are less likely to attend to preventive and other innovative efforts or to involve other health care professionals in team efforts (Mechanic, 1999:154-155).

Provider Service Organizations

One of the newest HMO types is the provider service organization. According to Rovner (1998):

> PSOs resemble HMOs in that they require patients to receive care from the plan's own doctors and hospitals, and patients must agree to have their care "managed" by the plan. The difference between a PSO and other plans is that a PSO offers its services through the doctors and hospitals who are owners of the PSO. (2)

Dick Davidson, President of the American Hospital Association, refers to PSOs as "community care networks" and apparently views them as a potential solution to the reduction in hospital inpatient usage in recent years and the reduction in hospital income resulting from managed care organization efforts to reduce health care costs by reducing hospital rates. Davidson advocates for PSOs partly because he sees them as having the advantage of local control over vertically integrated health care systems rather than control by huge HMO corporations often located in some other state (Grayson, 1998).

Preferred Provider Organizations

A related type of health care organization is the preferred provider organization, which is not really a form of HMO, but instead simply means that the insuring organization, such as Blue Shield, contracts with a network of physicians and other health service providers to provide services at a discounted price. Presumably, it is not considered a form of HMO because it remains a fee-for-service system, but one in which the fees are contracted at reduced amounts.

Point-of-Service

"Point of service" is a provision that may be associated with any of the HMO models and simply means that the model provides for patients having the choice to utilize health care providers outside the HMO, with the understanding that they must pay extra out of pocket for such outside services.

In other words, as Kovner (1999) noted:

> Managed care organizations are health care systems under which a broad scope of medical services is provided for a fixed amount of money, negotiated in advance . . . and health maintenance organizations are [but] one model of managed care. (280)

According to Kovner (1999):

> what differentiates HMOs [not all managed care organizations] from traditional health care delivery are the following factors: (1) the combining of the financing and delivery systems under a single organizational entity; (2) a broad scope of benefits; (3) a voluntarily enrolled population (unless the employer offers no alternative plan to the employees); (4) prepayment; (5) an organized provider system; and (6) the assumption of financial risk by the HMO. (282)

Kovner (1999:285) identifies "five main elements of HMOs: *purchasers, plans, hospital providers, medical providers, and members*":

1. The *purchaser* is an employer seeking a health care coverage plan for his or her employees, who prepays the "plan" for coverage of the enrolled employees.
2. The *members* are the employees enrolled in the plan.
3. The *plan* is both the contract itself and the organization that contracts with the purchaser, which may or may not be the same as the provider.
4. The *hospital provider* is either owned by the plan organization or contracts with it to provide needed hospital services to members referred by their HMO physician.
5. The *physician providers* are related to the *plan* under either the IPA (independent practice association model), the Group Model, or the Staff Model. (285-286)

Many HMO *plans* are owned by insurance companies, but they are also owned by cooperatives, nonprofit organizations, hospitals, and doctor groups (Kovner, 1999:284).

Trends and Impacts of Managed Care

Since the 1970s, managed care organizations have tended to shift from predominately nonprofit to predominately for-profit organizations with stockholder ownership. Furthermore, the theory behind the original health maintenance organization was that by focusing on primary and preventive care, health care costs could be controlled by reducing the need for more costly repair services from specialists (Mechanic, 1999:155). By shifting from a fee-for-service system to a prepaid service system, a mechanism of financial incentive was provided to physicians and other providers to focus on "health maintenance" (Mizrahi, 1993).

Today, however, managed care seems little involved in "preventive care" (Munson, 1997) and more involved in preventing physicians and other health service providers from using interventions that are not established by outcomes research as cost-effective. This change in the direction of HMOs has important implications for the concept of "professional" and tends to shift the focus of professional services from the provider-patient relationship and its alleged healing power as a medium of intervention (Munson, 1997; Schuster et al., 1994) to a focus on the independent efficacy of a particular technological intervention, such as a drug, surgical procedure, or form of psychotherapy.

The introduction of "managed care" also impacts on the meaning of a "professional" because a key ingredient in this concept has long been that a professional must be able to practice with relative *autonomy*. If, instead, third-party bureaucrats, with little or no education or training in the field of practice in question, are empowered to refer to computer-recorded protocols for the preferred procedure for treating a particular health problem—and to approve or deny a professional health care provider's intervention plan—professional autonomy, as traditionally conceptualized, is evidently lost (Munson, 1997).

As Cornelius (1994) noted, "In essence, the social worker becomes an agent of managed care and agrees to serve the public within the corporate guidelines and not necessarily according to the assessed needs of the client" (52). Strom-Gottfried (1998a) has expressed concern about the potential barriers imposed by managed care on the obligation of the professional provider to assure clients of the confidentiality of information concerning them, as well as to ensure that all interventions with clients and releases of information are preceded by obtaining their "informed consent."

A recent study by Chambliss, Pinto, and McGuigan (1997) found that among 139 mental health care professionals responding to a questionnaire sent to a randomly selected sample of 200 such professionals, considerable concern was expressed about perceived diminished client confidentiality and harmful effects on clients as a result of utilization reviews (149). Davidson and Davidson (1996) noted that "A document containing highly confidential material, in the hands of a managed care administrator, will be used whatever way is most profitable from a business perspective" (209). Concerning the issue of informed consent, reportedly, social work providers often feel compelled to get their clients to sign release of information forms in order to get reimbursed, while knowing that the clients' clinical information may be misused (Davidson and Davidson, 1996).

Strom-Gottfried (1998b) has proposed that it may be possible to resolve many of the current conflicts between providers and case managers in utilization review organizations through applying mediation techniques. Citing Moore (1986), Strom-Gottfried (1998b) lists the common sources of such disputes as including: "inconsistencies in data; relationship issues; value conflicts; structural problems such as unequal power or resources or geographic or physical barriers; and conflicts about interests" and makes the interesting observation that ". . . a primary principle in conflict resolution is to focus on interests, broadly defined, rather than positions" (395).

In a sense, proprietary managed care organizations are the current answer of the free-market health insurance industry to the perceived threat to itself of a single-payer plan, such as national health insurance or a national health service, or other government intervention as a mechanism of controlling health care costs.

"The HMO's response to traditional indemnity financing is offer a price to the purchaser of only 80 percent of the traditional price and at the same time achieve a bottom line profit that is 50 percent greater than that of the traditional indemnity insurer" (Hodge, 1996, cited in Kovner, 1999:297). This private reduction typically comes from three sources—reductions of about one-third each in payments to specialists, drug suppliers, and hospitals (Kovner, 1999:297).

Some HMO executives have made as much as $10 million a year in salary and bonuses and much more than that as a result of increases in the stock prices of the HMO (Kovner, 1999:299). The for-profits have been growing rapidly, in large part because of their advantages over nonprofits in securing large amounts of capital (Kovner, 1999:284).

Commenting on the current market-driven takeover of the U.S. health care system, Robert B. Friedland (1996), Director of the National Academy on Aging, predicts:

> . . . in about twenty years, what was once a market-based evolution will become a state-based public enterprise. Managed care will still be with us, but so too will managed financing, as state utility commissions set the rates and the policies concerning the care provided by the publicly regulated health plans. (41)

SUMMARY

The *strengths* of the U.S. health care system include a generally high quality of medical care and highly advanced technological interventions to repair and manage health problems. In addition, there are generally high standards, both legal and professional, for the training and practice of physicians and other health and allied health professionals in the United States. Although often critical of the nation's health care system, most Americans are quite satisfied with their own health care services.

On the other hand, there are significant *problems* with the U.S. health care system, including the fact that the health status indicators of the population do not sufficiently reflect the proportion of our economic resources that we expend for health care. Presumably, this is the result of our tendency to focus on the acute level of health care, with comparatively little in the way of supportive interventions to (1) prevent the occurrence of health problems, (2) intervene early to prevent their development, or (3) provide supportive interventions to maximize the comfort and function of those with chronic or terminal impairments. In other words, we are preoccupied with "curing" to the neglect of "caring," at all levels of health service.

We also tend to "overuse" diagnostic and repair technology in the sense that health care providers often use it even when its cost-effectiveness is not well established. We have come to equate "doing something" with the diagnosis and repair of health problems and have sometimes lost sight of the things one can "do" to prevent their occurrence, development, and unnecessary effects that impair comfort and function.

The major value of managed care would be realized if it reduced waste in the health care system without reducing the quality of care. We need to reexamine our tendency in America to think of specialization and high technology as "sexy" and to think of generalist practice, primary care, and long-term care as dull and unchallenging.

Some trends in our health care system hold promise, I think, such as the move toward greater continuity of health care via vertically integrated health care systems, greater concentration of resources on primary care, more attention to outcomes research as criteria for intervention planning, and setting limits on available resources to pay for health care and forcing providers to think more about the cost-effectiveness of intervention options.

On the other hand, some of us question the morality of CEOs of profit-making managed care organizations being rewarded with multimillion dollar annual salaries and benefits packages in a nation where about 40 million citizens have no health insurance, and millions more must regularly choose between groceries or uncovered health care needs. Here the issue is *equity*, that is, *what is fair or just*. Furthermore, it does seem to make sense that a single-payer system such as Canada's would likely reduce the current administrative costs in the United States of having multiple insurance organizations. For one thing, a single-payer system under national health insurance eliminates "bad debts" and so reduces provider overhead costs, which currently get shifted to the fees of those who do pay (Belcher, 1993). Canadian hospitals receive an annual global budget at the beginning of each year and must operate within it; they also do not have the expense of filing claims for reimbursement, as they have already been funded for the year, adding to administrative cost savings.

What we need, I think, are more HMOs of the Kaiser Permanente kind—nonprofit, with health care providers who make their own decisions about choice of interventions and themselves assume the financial risk of exceeding the capitated prepayment, and within which considerable interprofessional teamwork is the norm, including efforts at health education and health behavior modification.

Chapter 9

A Vision of Future
Social Work Practice in Health Care

INTRODUCTION

This final chapter concerns reflections on the past and future of social work in the health field, the need for social policy changes that will promote better health *care* at all levels of intervention— prevention, remediation, and compensation—and the need for out- comes research to further develop a body of social work practice knowledge in the field.

EMERGING TRENDS
IN HEALTH CARE DELIVERY

Among the changes occurring in the United States that impact on the future of social work in the health field are the following: (1) the shift from the hospital to the community as the center of health care delivery; (2) the increase in health problems with social and envi- ronmental etiology; (3) the public demand for more input into per- sonal health care decisions, in the context of increasing complex medical and surgical intervention options; (4) the growing expecta- tion that families will have to do more of the caregiving of their own members, at all levels of caring; (5) the gradual transformation of once-terminal health problems into more chronic long-term care ones; and (6) the interaction of profit-oriented managed care and its principles with these changes (Vaghy, 1998:8).

In addition, there is growing recognition of the importance of health promotion and health problem prevention, coupled with payer demands for efficiency and cost-effectiveness, outcomes documentation, quality management and improvement mechanisms, and integration of patient-focused service provision across professional boundaries (Spitzer and Nash, 1996).

IMPLICATIONS

The following paradigm shifts in health care have implications for future social work practice in the health field: from institution-based to community-based care, from directive to supportive care, from a medical or disease focus to a health and prevention focus, from a passive patient and family to an active participating patient and family, and from episodic care to continuity of care (Volland, 1996:47).

Furthermore, social workers in health care settings are faced with a need for clinical intervention in patient health care education, ethical practice dilemmas, greater consumer diversity, need for more social work research, and the need to reexamine what social workers do in health care (Browne et al., 1996).

Another, not insignificant change that has impacted social work practice is the replacement of traditional social worker clinical supervision with oversight by staff of managed care organizations, who have little or no clinical training, yet usually shift the legal and ethical responsibility to the clinician (Munson, 1998:315).

Also, there is undeniable evidence of the interdependence of biological, psychological, and social environmental phenomena. Accordingly, the dubious distinction that lingers between "physical" and "mental" health arenas needs to be reconsidered.

The Need for Social Work to Develop a Body of Practice Research

For years, the call has been going out in the social work in health care literature for social workers to "demonstrate their effectiveness" if they hope to retain their positions in the field. Unfortunately, this call for outcomes research has not been sufficiently heeded. Now there is growing evidence that social work is not widely recognized as a key health care profession (Rosenberg, 1998:9-10).

Rosenberg (1998) points to the following factors as some of the barriers to social work being accorded a firm position in the health field: its association with a relatively powerless "welfare" clientele; its presence as some competition with physicians; its failure to demonstrate the cost-effectiveness of its services; its being seen as ineffective in resolving social problems (which require the cooperation of powers beyond social work alone); its lack of outcome data to develop "best practices," as well as its failure to employ quality management processes; its lack of effective collaboration with other health care professionals to address social health problems; and its lack of a "track record" of work to improve public social health policy (12). In short:

> Interventions are needed to address [health] behavior and to promote the creation and maintenance of social support. . . . The need is growing for social work to step back from health care, aging, disability, mental health, and managed care and to reconceptualize its roles in the entire dynamic holistic continuum of care and services: prevention, health promotion, service delivery design, acute and chronic care, treatment, rehabilitation, and long-term care. (Keigher, 1997:151)

Volland (1996) warns that "The results of outcome management studies will play an increasingly important role in determining the level and type of financial support a specific health care service [such as social work] will receive" (49).

Furthermore, managed care itself is such a dilemma for social workers that, as Veeder and Peebles-Wilkins (1998) noted:

> A commitment must be made to evaluate every aspect of managed care, from services delivered and their outcomes, to administrative issues, to ethical concerns, to policies generated and implemented, to protocol proprietorship and other legal and statutory issues, and to the comparative viability of managed care approaches to behavioral health care. (489)

Some Tools for Outcomes Research

In response to the increased demand for outcomes research and documentation of diagnostic accuracy and intervention effectiveness at the primary care level, Van Hook, Berkman, and Dunkle

(1996) have proposed that social workers in primary care settings make increased use of some of the existing instruments appropriate to (1) mental health problem assessment, such as PRIME-MD; (2) the functional assessment of older persons, such as OARS; and (3) assessment of the health-related quality of life, such as the HRQL instrument (SF-36).

PRIME-MD (Primary Care Evaluation of Mental Health Disorders) targets (1) mood, (2) anxiety, (3) somataform disorders, (4) eating disorders, and (5) alcohol abuse and facilitates identification of any of eighteen common diagnostic categories of the DSM-IV (Van Hook, Berkman, and Dunkle, 1996).

The OARS questionnaire (Older Americans Resources Survey) is instrumental in assessing older persons' level of ability to perform activities of daily living (ADLs) and instrumental ADLs, in addition to their social resources, economic resources, mental health and physical health. It also "can be used for screening, evaluating outcomes, and modeling the cost-effectiveness of alternative approaches of care" (McDowell and Newell, 1987, cited in Van Hook, Berkman, and Dunkle, 1996:231).

Finally, the SF-36 instrument focuses on Health-Related Quality of Life (HRQL) indicators, from a patient's perspective. Essentially, it addresses issues of the impact of physical or mental health problems on ability to perform physical activities, usual roles, social activities, mental health and well-being, energy level, and perceptions of overall health. An advantage of the tool is that it can be completed by clients age fourteen or older in ten minutes or less. It is currently believed to be most appropriately used in measuring outcomes at a group level and has yet to be assessed in terms of use at the individual level (Van Hook, Berkman, and Dunkle, 1996; Berkman, 1998).

Davis (1998:417) wrote, "Clinical practice in managed care emphasizes a short-term, problem-focused acute care model based in part on measurement scales designed to aid in diagnosis and outcome assessment."

Curing and Caring

As was stated in the preface, professionals in health care need to expand the focus of their attention from preoccupation with repairing human problems (curing) to a more *supportive* approach to helping (caring) at each level of health intervention: (1) prevention, (2) remediation of early problems, and (3) compensation for chronic or terminal health problems.

Need for a Technology of Caring

As David Mechanic advised over twenty years ago, we need to develop a "technology of caring" to more effectively address the chronic and psychosocial health problems that predominate today (Mechanic, 1978).

Davidson (1998), citing Monkman (1991) and Ell (1996), wrote:

> . . . the psychosocial arena is too often perceived as everyone's area of expertise. It remains imperative for social workers to demonstrate through research studies that the professional expertise that allows us to provide *supportive services* to families provides positive and welcome results, such as reduction of lost work or school days; decreased stress-induced illness; and fewer of the medical crises that are often related to lack of knowledge, non-compliance with treatment, and overburdened caretakers. Research can then be used to advocate for provision of psychosocial services throughout health care programs. (426)

The Etiological Role of Psychosocial Factors

Most of the health problems we face today are significantly caused by destructive human behavior or by ignorance, unrelieved environmental stress, social injustice, and other social or emotional conditions that are the arena of social workers more than physicians. Some common biopsychosocial problems that social workers can help to address include drug and alcohol abuse, child abuse and neglect, domestic violence, elder abuse, teenage pregnancy, sexually transmitted diseases, suicide, depression, homicide, motor vehicle accidents, tobacco addiction, eating disorders, obsessive-compulsive behaviors, panic disorders, agoraphobia, social isolation, emotional withdrawal, and self-mutilation behavior.

The Mediating Role of Social Support

Perhaps the strongest argument for professional social workers playing a major role in health care in the future is the evidence that mediating structures, such as social support, *are the most powerful determinant of health.* The key role of such community support in promoting a healthy society cannot be overemphasized (Kelner, 1985).

CONCLUSION

Essentially, we need to develop a repertoire of effective supportive interventions to address the needs of the aged and others with chronic impairments, as well as those who are temporarily impaired, terminally ill, or need supportive assistance to prevent impairment—such as those whose lifestyle is reckless, as well as those who simply need care to grow and develop. The key to effective caring is to relieve "helplessness," assessed objectively and subjectively, by both the helper and the one who needs caring.

Caring is attending to the needs of a person that extend beyond the correction or control of an existing health condition or other type of problem. These needs may relate to prevention of such problems, to support of function or comfort during a problem episode, or to adjustment, adaption, or compensation for an incurable problem. Caring refers to interventions aimed at strengthening the ability of another person to cope with the impairing effect of any condition, situation, or event—whether childhood, old age, illness or injury, loss of a loved one, loss of employment, or a natural disaster.

In summary, whether the supports are interpersonal or concrete, the essence of care or caring is to strengthen the ability of people to cope with their impairment, to help people who need supportive assistance to save them from distress so they can have an improved quality of life. Such distress may result from the inability to sustain comfort, function, growth and development, or protection from harm. Caring is the way we relieve the distress of such impairment.

Supportive care interventions are empowering. They help to strengthen a person's ability to cope with an impairing condition, whether age, illness, injury, or other loss. Caring enables the person to have an easier path. It supplements and strengthens the powers of the victim. Caring helps to sustain the quality of life and to prevent or relieve distress.

Perhaps social work should take the lead in drawing representatives of other relevant groups into an interdisciplinary proposal for foundation funding to establish an Institute for Research and Development of Care Technology. This center would house, for example, architects, engineers, nurses, occupational therapists, patients, physicians, physical therapists, social workers, speech therapists, sociologists, economists, and medical anthropologists, who would together identify current dilemmas in the health care field, prioritize them, and form interdisciplinary work groups to jointly develop efficacious interventions to address them. Such work and products would constitute a new "science of caring."

References

Chapter 1

American Hospital Association (1997). AHA annual survey data faxed to the author on August 15, 1997, by Mark Barbaree, AHA Resources Center, Chicago, Illinois.

Bope, Edward T. and Jost, Timothy S. (1994). Interprofessional collaboration: Factors that affect form, function, and structure. In Casto, R. Michael, Julia, Maria C., Platt, Larry J., Harbaugh, Gary L., Waugaman, Wynne R., Thompson, Arlene, Jost, Timothy S., Bope, Edward T., Williams, Tennyson, and Lee, Daniel B. *Interprofessional care and collaborative practice.* Pacific Grove, CA: Brooks-Cole, 61-69.

Bracht, Neil F. (1978). *Social work in health care: A guide to professional practice.* Binghamton, NY: The Haworth Press, Inc.

Briggs, Margaret H. (1997). *Building early intervention teams.* Gaithersburg, MD: Aspen Publications.

Bucher, Rue and Stelling, Joan (1978). Characteristics of professional organizations. In Swartz, Howard D. and Kart, Cary S. (Eds.), *Dominant issues in medical sociology.* Reading, MA: Addison-Wesley, 340-351.

Cabot, Richard C. (1928). Hospital and dispensary social work. In Goldstine, Dora (Ed.) (1955), *Expanding horizons in medical social work.* Chicago: University of Chicago Press, 255-270.

Cannon, Ida M. (1923). *Social work in hospitals.* New York: Russell Sage.

Caputi, Marie A. (1978). Social work in health care: Past and future. *Health and Social Work,* 3(1): 9-29.

Casto, R. Michael (1994). Education for interprofessional practice. In Casto, R. Michael, Julia, Maria C., Platt, Larry J., Harbaugh, Gary L., Waugaman, Wynne R., Thompson, Arlene, Jost, Timothy S., Bope, Edward T., Williams, Tennyson, and Lee, Daniel B. *Interprofessional care and collaborative practice.* Pacific Grove, CA: Brooks-Cole, 95-110

Coe, R. (1978). *Sociology of medicine.* New York: McGraw-Hill.

Cowles, Lois A. (1990). Medical social work in hospitals: Interdisciplinary expectations of the role. Unpublished doctoral dissertation. University of Wisconsin Library, Madison. University Microfilms No. 9020434.

Cowles, Lois A. and Lefcowitz, Myron J. (1995). Interdisciplinary expectations of the medical social worker in the hospital setting: Part 2. *Health and Social Work,* 20(4): 279-286.

Engel, George L. (1977). The need for a new medical model: A challenge for biomedicine. *Science*, 196: 129-136.

French, Ruth (1979). *Dynamics of health care*. New York: McGraw Hill.

Friedson, Elliot (1978). The prospects for health services in the U.S. *Medical Care*, 16(12): 971-983.

Gibelman, Margaret and Schervish, Phillip H. (1996). *Who we are*. Washington, DC: NASW Press.

Ginsberg, Leon (1995). *The social work almanac* (Second edition). Washington, DC: NASW Press.

Given, Barbara and Simmons, Sandra (1977). The interdisciplinary health care team: Fact or fiction. *Nursing Forum*, 16(2): 165-177.

Goffman, Erving (1961). *Asylums: Essays on the social situation of mental patients and other inmates*. Garden City, NJ: Doubleday.

Grob, Gerald N. (1983). *Mental illness and American society: 1875-1940*. Princeton, NJ: Princeton University Press.

Harris, J.W., Saunders, D.N., and Zasorin-Conners, J. (1978). A training program for interprofessional health care teams. *Health and Social Work*, 3(2): 35-53.

Jonas, Steve (1981). *Health care delivery in the United States*. New York: Springer.

Julia, Maria C. and Thompson, Arlene (1994a). Group process and interprofessional teamwork. In Casto, R. Michael, Julia, Maria C., Platt, Larry J., Harbaugh, Gary L., Waugaman, Wynne R., Thompson, Arlene, Jost, Timothy S., Bope, Edward T., Williams, Tennyson, and Lee, Daniel B. *Interprofessional care and collaborative practice*. Pacific Grove, CA: Brooks-Cole, 35-42.

Julia, Maria C. and Thompson, Arlene (1994b). Essential elements of interprofessional teamwork. In Casto, R. Michael, Julia, Maria C., Platt, Larry J., Harbaugh, Gary L., Waugaman, Wynne R., Thompson, Arlene, Jost, Timothy S., Bope, Edward T., Williams, Tennyson, and Lee, Daniel B. *Interprofessional care and collaborative practice*. Pacific Grove, CA: Brooks-Cole, 43-58.

Kane, Rosalie (1976-1977). Interprofessional education and social work: A survey. *Social Work in Health Care*, 2(2): 229-238.

Kane, Rosalie (1978). The interprofessional team as a small group. In Bracht, Neil (Ed.), *Social work in health care: A guide to professional practice*. Binghamton, NY: The Haworth Press, Inc., 85-97.

Kane, Rosalie (1980). Multidisciplinary teamwork in the U.S.: trends, issues, and implications for the social worker. In Lonsdale, Susan, Webb, Adrian, and Briggs, Thomas L. (Eds.), *Teamwork in the personal social services and health care*. Syracuse, NY: Syracuse University School of Social Work, 138-151.

Karger, Howard Jacob and Stoesz, David (1994). *American social welfare policy: A pluralist approach* (Second edition). New York: Longman.

Karger, Howard Jacob and Stoesz, David (1998). *American social welfare policy: A pluralist approach* (Third edition). New York: Longman.

Levy, Norman B. (1974). The giving-up-given-up complex. In Simons, Richard C. and Pardes, Herbert (Eds.), *Understanding human behavior in health and illness*. Baltimore, MD: Williams and Wilkins, 430-435.

Lodge, Richard (1974). University education in interprofessional perspectives. In Rehr, Helen (Ed.), *Medicine and social work: An exploration of interprofessionalism*, New York: Prodist, 26-32.

Lonsdale, Susan, Webb, Adrian, and Briggs, Thomas L. (Eds.) (1980). *Teamwork in the personal social services and health care*. Syracuse, NY: Syracuse University School of Social Work.

Lubove, Roy (1965). *The professional altruist: The emergence of social work as a career*. Cambridge, MA: Harvard University Press.

Mailick, Mildred D. and Jordon, Pearl (1977). A multimodal approach to collaborative practice in health settings. *Social Work in Health Care*, 2(4): 445-454.

McLachlan, Gordon and McKeown, Thomas (Eds.) (1971). *Medical history and medical care*. London: Oxford University Press.

Nagi, Saad Z. (1978). Teamwork in health care in the U.S.: A sociological perspective. In Schwartz, Howard D. and Kart, Cary S. (Eds.), *Dominant issues in medical sociology*. Reading, MA: Addison-Wesley, 490-498.

National Association of Social Workers (1983). Membership survey data obtained through phone conversation with an NASW research associate during Summer 1992.

National Association of Social Workers (1987). NASW standards for social work in health care settings. Washington, DC: NASW Press, 30 pp.

Platt, Larry J. (1994). Why bother with teams: An overview. In Casto, R. Michael, Julia, Maria C., Platt, Larry J., Harbaugh, Gary L., Waugaman, Wynne R., Thompson, Arlene, Jost, Timothy S., Bope, Edward T., Williams, Tennyson, and Lee, Daniel B. *Interprofessional care and collaborative practice*. Pacific Grove, CA: Brooks-Cole, 3-10.

Popple, Philip R. and Leighninger, Leslie (1993). *Social work, social welfare, and American society* (Second edition). Boston, MA: Allyn and Bacon.

Rubin, Irwin M. and Beckhard, Richard (1972). Factors influencing the effectiveness of health teams. *Milbank Memorial Fund Quarterly*, 50 (Part 1): 317-335.

Schmale, Arthur H. (1972). Giving up as a final common pathway to changes in health. *Advances in Psychosomatic Medicine*, 8: 20-40.

Sheps, Cecil G. (1974). Developmental perspectives on interprofessional education. In Rehr, Helen (Ed.), *Medicine and social work: An exploration of interprofessionalism*. New York: Prodist., 3-13.

Smith, Harvey L. (1978). Two lines of authority: The hospitals' dilemma. In Swartz, Howard D. and Kart, Cary S. (Eds.), *Dominant issues in medical sociology*. Reading, MA: Addison-Wesley, 315-322.

Stuart, Paul H. (1997). Community care and the origins of psychiatric social work. *Social Work in Health Care*, 25(3): 25-36.

Trattner, Walter I. (1989). *From poor law to welfare state: A history of social welfare in America* (Fourth edition). New York: The Free Press.

Waugaman, Wynne R. (1994). Professionalization and socialization in interprofessional collaboration. In Casto, R. Michael, Julia, Maria C., Platt, Larry J., Harbaugh, Gary L., Waugaman, Wynne R., Thompson, Arlene, Jost, Timothy S.,

Bope, Edward T., Williams, Tennyson, and Lee, Daniel B. *Interprofessional care and collaborative practice.* Pacific Grove, CA: Brooks-Cole, 23-32.

World Health Organization (1978). *Alma-Ata 1978: Primary health care—Report of the international conference on primary health care.* Alma-Ata, Union of Soviet Socialist Republics. 6-12. September 1978. Geneva: WHO.

Chapter 2

Blazyk, Stan and Canavan, Margaret (1985). Therapeutic aspects of discharge planning. *Social Work,* 30(6): 489-496.

DiNitto, Diana M. and McNeece, C. Aaron (1997). *Social work: Issues and opportunities in a challenging profession* (Second edition). Boston, MA: Allyn and Bacon.

Germain, Carel B. and Gitterman, Alex (1980). *The life model of social work practice.* New York: Columbia University Press.

Goffman, Erving (1961). *Asylums: Essays on the social situation of mental patients and other inmates.* Garden City, NJ: Doubleday.

Greenwood, Ernest (1957). Attributes of a profession. *Social Work,* 2(3) (July): 45-55.

Kerson, Toba Schwaber (1989). *Social work in health settings: Practice in context.* Binghamton, NY: The Haworth Press.

Levy, Norman B. (1974). The giving-up-given-up complex. In Simons, Richard C. and Pardes, Herbert (Eds.), *Understanding human behavior in health and illness.* Baltimore, MD: Williams and Wilkins.

McLachlan, Gordon and McKeown, Thomas (Eds.) (1971). *Medical history and medical care.* London: Oxford University Press.

McKeown, Thomas (1979). *The role of medicine: Dream, mirage, or nemesis.* London: Blackwell Press.

Mechanic, David (1978). *Medical sociology.* New York: The Free Press.

Morales, Armando and Sheafor, Bradford (1989). *Social work: A profession of many faces.* Boston, MA: Allyn and Bacon.

Morris, Robert and Anderson, Delwin (1975). Personal care services: An identity for social work. *Social Service Review,* 41(2): 157-174.

National Association of Social Workers (1987). NASW standards for social work in health care settings. Washington, DC: NASW Press.

National Association of Social Workers (1991). *The social work dictionary.* Washington, DC: NASW Press.

National Association of Social Workers (1996). NASW code of ethics. Washington, DC: NASW Press.

Neuman, W. Lawrence (1994). *Social research methods: Qualitative and quantitative approaches.* Boston, MA: Allyn and Bacon.

Schmale, Arthur H. (1972). Giving up as a final common pathway to changes in health. *Advances in Psychosomatic Medicine,* 8: 20-40.

Seligman, Martin E. (1975). *Helplessness.* San Francisco, CA: W.H. Freeman and Co.

Wing, John W. (1978). *Reasoning about madness.* Oxford, England: Oxford Press.

World Health Organization (1978). *Alma-Ata 1978: Primary health care: Report of the international conference on primary health care.* Alma-Ata, Union of Soviet Socialist Republics. 6-12. September 1978. Geneva: WHO.

Chapter 3

Badger, Lee W., Ackerson, Barry, Buttell, Frederick, and Rand, Elizabeth H. (1997). The case for integration of social work psychosocial services into rural primary care practice. *Health and Social Work,* 22(1): 20-29.

Bloom, Martin (1987). Prevention. In Minahan, Anne (Ed.), *The Encyclopedia of Social Work* (Eighteenth edition). Washington, DC: NASW Press, 303-311.

Bloom, Martin (1995). Primary prevention overview. In Edwards, Richard L. (Ed.), *The Encyclopedia of Social Work.* Washington, DC: NASW Press, 1895-1904.

Bracht, Neil (Ed.) (1990). *Health promotion at the community level.* Thousand Oaks, CA: Sage Publications.

Cabot, Richard C. (1955). Hospital and dispensary social work. In Goldstine, D. (Ed.), *Expanding horizons in medical social work.* Chicago: University of Chicago Press, 255-270.

Cannon, Ida M. (1923). *Social work in hospitals.* New York: Russell Sage.

Cassell, Eric (1995). Teaching the fundamentals of primary care: A point of view. *The Milbank Quarterly,* 75(3): 373-405.

Clare, Anthony W. (1982). Social aspects of ill-health in general practice. In Clare, Anthony W. and Corney, Roslyn H. (Eds.), *Social work and primary health care.* London: Academic Press, 9-22.

Cleveland, Tessie (1981). Where are we going with specialty interest groups? *Health and Social Work,* 6(4): 9s-12s.

Cockerham, William C. (1992). *Medical sociology.* Englewood Cliffs, NJ: Prentice-Hall.

Corin, Ellen E. (1994). The social and cultural matrix of health and disease. In Evans, Robert G., Barer, Morris L., and Marmor, Theodore R. (Eds.), *Why are some people healthy and others not? The determinants of health of populations.* New York: Aldine De Gruyter.

Cowles, Lois A. and Lefcowitz, Myron J. (1995). Interdisciplinary expectations of the medical social worker in the hospital setting: Part 2. *Health and Social Work,* 20(4): 279-286.

Davis, King E. (1996). Primary health care and severe mental illness: The need for national and state policy. *Health and Social Work,* 21(2): 83-87.

Dobrof, Judith, Umpierre, Mari, Rocha, Loraine, and Silverton, Marsha (1990). Group work in a primary care medical setting. *Health and Social Work,* 15(1): 32-37.

Donaldson, Molla S., Yordy, Karl D., Lohr, Kathleen N., and Vanselow, Neal A. (Eds.) (1996). *Primary care: America's health in a new era.* Washington, DC: National Academy Press.

Dunlop, Judith and Holosko, Michael (1992). Community social work practice: Health promotion in action. In Holosko, Michael J. and Taylor, Patricia A.

(Eds.), *Social work practice in health settings* (Second edition). Toronto, Canada: Canadian Scholar's Press, 643-656.

Ell, Kathleen, and Morrison, Diane R. (1981). Primary care. *Health and Social Work*, 6(4) (supplement): 35s-43s.

Engel, George (1977). The need for a new medical model: A challenge for biomedicine. *Science*, 196: 129-136.

Evans, Robert G., Barer, Morris L., and Marmor, Theodore R. (Eds.) (1994). *Why are some people healthy and others not? The determinants of health of populations.* New York: Aldine De Gruyter.

Freund, Peter E.S. and McGuire, Meridith B. (1991). *Health, illness, and the social body: A critical sociology.* Englewood Cliffs, NJ: Prentice-Hall.

Friis, Robert H. and Sellers, Thomas A. (1996). *Epidemiology for public health practice.* Gaithersburg, MD: Aspen Publishers.

Green, Gilbert J. and Kulper, Teresa (1990). Autonomy and professional activities of social workers in hospital and primary health care settings. *Health and Social Work*, 15(1)(February): 38-44.

Green, James W. (1995). *Cultural awareness in the human services: A multi-ethnic approach* (Second edition). Boston, MA: Allyn and Bacon.

Gross, Revital, Rabinowitz, Johnothan, Feldman, Dina, and Boerma, Wienke (1996). Primary health care physician's treatment of psychosocial problems. *Health and Social Work*, 21(2): 174-181.

Gullotta, T.P. (1987). Prevention's technology. *Journal of Primary Prevention,* 8(1): 4-24.

Henk, Mat L. (1989). *Social work in primary care.* Thousand Oaks, CA: Sage.

Hess, Howard (1985). Social work clinical practice in family medicine centers: The need for a practice model. *Journal of Social Work Education,* 21(1): 56-65. (Quoted material reprinted with permission of the Council on Social Work Education, Department of Sociology, Social Work, and Criminal Justice, 1600 Duke Street, Alexandria, VA.)

Hill, Dana Robin, Kelleher, K., and Shumaker, Sally A. (1992). Psychosocial interventions in adult patients with coronary heart disease and cancer: A literature review. *General Hospital Psychiatry,* 145(65): 28s-42s.

Katon, Wayne (1987). The epidemiology of depression in medical care. *International Journal of Psychiatry in Medicine,* 17(1): 93-112.

Katon, Wayne and Schulberg, Herbert (1992). Epidemiology of depression in primary care. *General Hospital Psychiatry,* 14(4)(Supplement 6): 237-247.

Kelner, M. (1985). Community support networks: Current issues. *Canadian Journal of Public Health,* 76 (supplement 1): 69-70.

Kerson, Toba Schwaber and Peachey, Helen (1989). Family planning agency: An unsuccessful contraceptor. In Kerson, Toba Schwaber (Ed.), *Social work in health settings: Practice in context,* Binghamton, NY: The Haworth Press, Inc., 231-245.

Kozol, Jonathan (1991). *Savage inequalities: Children in America's schools.* New York: HarperCollins.

Kozol, Jonathan (1995). *Amazing grace: The lives of children and the conscience of a nation.* New York: Crown Publishing Group.

Marshack, Elaine, Davidson, Kay, and Mizrahi, Terry (1988). Preparation of social workers for a changing health care environment. *Health and Social Work,* 13(3)(Summer): 226-233.

Mechanic, David (1994). Integrating mental health into a general health care system. *Hospital and Community Psychiatry,* 45(9): 893-897.

Miller, Rosalind (1987). Primary health care. In Minahan, Anne (Ed.), *Encyclopedia of social work* (Eighteenth edition). Washington, DC: NASW Press.

National Association of Community Health Centers (1993). *National directory of community health centers, migrant health centers, health care for the homeless projects and primary care associations.* Washington, DC: Author.

National Association of Social Workers (1987). NASW standards for social work in health care settings. Washington, DC: NASW Press.

National Association of Social Workers (1996). NASW code of ethics. Washington, DC: NASW Press.

Oktay, Julianne S. (1984, March). Social workers in primary health care: A national study of tasks and functions. Presented at the CSWE Annual Program Meeting, Detroit, MI.

Oktay, Julianne S. (1995). Primary health care. In Edwards, Richard L. (Ed.), *The encyclopedia of social work* (Nineteenth edition). Washington, DC: NASW Press, 1887-1894.

Pert, Candace, Ruff, Michael, Weber, Richard, and Herkenham, Miles (1985). Neuropeptides and their receptors: A psychosomatic network. *Journal of Immunology,* 135 (Supplement 2): 820s-826s.

Pray, Kenneth (1995). Prevention and wellness. In Edwards, Richard L. (Ed.), *The encyclopedia of social work* (Nineteenth edition). Washington, DC: NASW Press, 1879-1886.

Shannon, Mary T. (1989). Health promotion and illness prevention: A biopsychosocial perspective. *Health and Social Work,* 14(1): 32-40.

Siefert, Kristine, Jayaratne, Srinika, and Martin, Louise Doss (1992). Implementing the public health social work forward plan: A research-based prevention curriculum for schools of social work. *Health and Social Work,* 17(1): 17-27.

Smyre, Patricia (1993). *Women and health.* London and Atlantic Highlands, NJ: Zed Books.

Trattner, Walter I. (1989). *From poor law to welfare state: A history of social welfare in America* (Fourth edition). New York: The Free Press.

Weiss, Gregory L. and Lonnquist, Lynne E. (1994). *The sociology of health, healing, and illness.* Englewood Cliffs, NJ: Prentice-Hall

Wheaton, Blair (1980). The sociogenesis of psychological disorder: An attributional theory. *Journal of Health and Social Behavior,* 21(2): 100-124.

Winslow, Charles-Edward Amory (1920). The untilled field of public health. *Modern Medicine,* 2(March): 183-191.

World Health Organization (1978). *Alma-Ata 1978: Primary health care: report of the international conference on primary health care*. Alma-Ata, Union of Soviet Socialist Republics. 6-12. September 1978. Geneva: WHO.

Young, Christine L. and Martin, Louise Doss (1989). Social services in rural and urban primary care projects. *Human Services in the Rural Environment*, 13(2): 30-35.

Zayas, Luis H. and Dyche, Larry A. (1992). Social workers training primary care physicians: Essential psychosocial principles. *Social Work*, 37(3): 247-252.

Chapter 4

Abramson, Julie S. (1990). Enhancing patient participation: Clinical strategies in the discharge planning process. *Social Work in Health Care*, 14(4): 53-70.

Abramson, Julie, Donnelly, James, King, Michael A., and Mailick, Mildred D. (1993). Disagreements in discharge planning: A normative phenomenon. *Health and Social Work*, 18(1): 57-64.

Abramson, Marcia (1996). Toward a more holistic understanding of ethics in social work. *Social Work in Health Care*, 23(2): 1-14.

American Hospital Association (1977). Development of professional standards review for hospital social work. Chicago, IL: Author, 28 pp.

American Hospital Association (1985). Phone conversation between author and an AHA spokesperson, Chicago, April.

American Hospital Association (1993/1994). American Hospital Association profile of United States hospitals. *AHA Hospital Statistics*. Chicago, IL: Author.

American Hospital Association (1997). AHA Resource Center, data derived from AHA *1995 Annual Survey*. Data faxed to author from Mark Barbaree.

Bartlett, Maria, C. and Baum, Bernard H. (1995). What happens to patients after nursing home placement? *Social Work in Health Care*, 22(1): 69-79.

Becker, Nancy E. and Becker, Fred W. (1986). Early identification of high social risk. *Health and Social Work*, 11(1): 26-35.

Beckerman, Nancy and Rock, Marjorie (1996). Themes from the frontlines: Hospital social work with people with AIDS. *Social Work in Health Care*, 23(4): 75-89.

Bennett, Claire, Legon, Julianne, and Zilberfein, Felice (1989). The significance of empathy in current hospital based practice. *Social Work in Health Care*, 14(2): 27-40.

Berger, Candyce S., Cayner, Jay, Mizrahi, Terry, Scesny, Alice, and Trachtenberg, Judith (1996). The changing scene of social work in hospitals. *Health and Social Work*, 21(3): 167-177.

Berkman, Barbara, Millar, Sally, Holmes, William, and Bonander, Evelyn (1991). Predicting elderly cardiac patients at risk for readmission. *Social Work in Health Care*, 16(1): 21-38.

Bloch, Linda von (1996). Breaking the bad news when sudden death occurs. *Social Work in Health Care*, 23(4): 91-97.

Cannon, Ida M. (1923). *Social work in hospitals*. New York: Russell Sage.

Caputi, Marie A. (1978). Social work in health care: Past and future. *Health and Social Work,* 3(1): 9-29.

Clemens, Elizabeth (1995). Multiple perceptions of discharge planning in one urban hospital. *Health and Social Work,* 20(4): 254-261.

Congress, Elaine P. and Lyons, Beverly P. (1992). Cultural differences in health beliefs: Implications for social work practice in health care settings. *Social Work in Health Care,* 17(3): 81-97.

Coulton, Claudia J. (1988). Evaluating screening and early intervention: A puzzle with many pieces. *Social Work in Health Care,* 13(3): 65-72.

Coulton, Claudia J. (1990). Research in patient and family decision making regarding life sustaining and long term care. *Social Work in Health Care,* 15(1): 63-78.

Coulton, Claudia J., Dunkle, Ruth E., Haug, Marie, Chow, Julian, and Vielhaber, David P. (1989). Locus of control and decision making for posthospital care. *The Gerontologist,* 29(5): 627-632.

Cowles, Lois A. and Lefcowitz, Myron J. (1992). Interdisciplinary expectations of the medical social worker in the hospital setting. *Health and Social Work,* 17(1): 57-65.

Cowles, Lois A. and Lefcowitz, Myron J. (1995). Interdisciplinary expectations of the medical social worker in the hospital setting: Part 2. *Health and Social Work,* 20(4): 279-286.

Cuzzi, Lawrence, Holden, Gary, Rutter, Steve, Rosenberg, Gary, and Chernack, Peter (1996). A pilot study of fieldwork rotations vs. year long placements for social work students in a public hospital. *Social Work in Health Care,* 24(1/2): 73-91.

Dobrof, Judith (1991). DRG's and the social worker's role in discharge planning. *Social Work in Health Care,* 16(2): 37-54.

Donnelly, James P. (1992). A frame for defining social work in a hospital setting. *Social Work in Health Care,* 18(1): 107-119.

Dubowitz, Howard, Black, Maureen, and Harrington, Donna (1992). The diagnosis of child sexual abuse. *American Journal of Diseases of Children,* 146(June): 688-693.

Egan, Marcia and Kadushin, Goldie (1995). Competitive allies: Rural nurses' and social workers' perceptions of the social work role in the hospital setting. *Social Work in Health Care,* 20(3): 1-23.

Evans, Ron L. and Connis, Richard T. (1996). Risk screening for adverse outcomes in subacute care. *Psychological Reports,* 78: 1043-1048.

Evans, Ron L., Hendricks, Robert D., Lawrence-Umlauf, Kaye V., and Bishop, Duane S. (1989). Timing of social work intervention and medical patients' length of hospital stay. *Health and Social Work,* 14(4)(November): 277-282.

Fahs, Marianne C. and Wade, Kathleen (1996). An economic analysis of two models of hospital care for AIDS patients: Implications for hospital discharge planning. *Social Work in Health Care,* 22(4): 21-34.

Feather, John (1993). Factors in perceived hospital discharge planning effectiveness. *Social Work in Health Care,* 19(1): 1-14.

Fillit, Howard, Howe, Judith L., Sachs, Charles, Sell, Laura, Siegel Patricia, Miller, Myron, and Butler, Robert N. (1992). Studies of hospital social stays in the frail elderly and their relationship to the intensity of social work intervention. *Social Work in Health Care*, 18(1): 1-22.

Foster, Larry W., Sharp, John, Scesny, Alice, McLellan, Linda, and Cotman, Kathy (1993). Bioethics: Social work's response and training needs. *Social Work in Health Care*, 19(1): 15-38.

Gentry, Linda R. (1993). Practice forum: The special caretakers program—A hospital's solution to the boarder baby problem. *Health and Social Work*, 18(1): 75-77.

Germain, Carel B. (1980). Social work identity, competence, and autonomy: The ecological perspective. *Social Work in Health Care*, 6(1): 1-10.

Ginsberg, Leon (1995). *The social work almanac* (Second edition). Washington, DC: NASW Press.

Glassman, Uania (1991). The social work group and its distinct healing qualities in the health care setting. *Health and Social Work*, 16(3): 203-212.

Globerman, Judith and Bogo, Marion (1995). Social work in the new integrative hospital. *Social Work in Health Care*, 21(3): 1-21.

Globerman, Judith, Davies, Joan MacKenzie, and Walsh, Susan (1996). Social work in restructuring hospitals: Meeting the challenge. *Health and Social Work*, 21(2): 178-188.

Hall, James A., Jensen, Greg V., Fortney, Mark A., Sutter, Joy, Locher, Jan, and Cayner, Jay J. (1996). Education of staff and students in health care settings: Integrating practice and research. *Social Work in Health Care*, 24(1/2): 93-113.

Hanson, James G. and Rapp, Charles A. (1992). Families' perceptions of community mental health programs for their relatives with a severe mental illness. *Community Mental Health Journal*, 28(3): 181-197.

Hanson, Meridith, Foreman, Lewis, Tomlin, Willie, and Bright, Yvonne (1994). Facilitating problem drinking clients' transition from inpatient to outpatient care. *Health and Social Work*, 19(1): 23-28.

Hazard, William R. (1995). Elder abuse: Definitions and implications for medical education. *Academic Medicine*, 70(11): 979-981.

Herbert, Margot and Levin, Ron (1996). The advocacy role in hospital social work. *Social Work in Health Care*, 22(3): 71-83.

James, Catherine D. and Studs, Dip Soc (1987). An ecological approach to defining discharge planning. *Social Work in Health Care*, 12(4): 47-59.

Julia, Maria C. (1996). *Multicultural awareness in the health care professions*. Boston, MA: Allyn and Bacon.

Kadushin, Goldie and Kulys, Regina (1995). Job satisfaction among social work discharge planners. *Health and Social Work*, 20(3): 174-186.

Keehn, Debra S., Roglitz, Cathy, and Bowden, M. Leora (1994). Impact of social work on recidivism and non-medical complaints in the emergency department. *Social Work in Health Care*, 20(1): 65-75.

Lauria, Marie M., Hockenberry-Eaton, Marilyn, Pawletko, Terese M., and Mauer, Alvin M. (1996). Psychosocial protocol for childhood cancer. *Cancer,* 78(6): 1345-1356.

Marcus, Leonard (1990). Research on organizational issues in health care social work. *Social Work in Health Care,* 15(1): 79-95.

Mayer, Jane B. (1995). The effective healthcare social work director: Managing the social work department at Beth Israel Hospital. *Social Work in Health Care,* 20(4): 61-72.

McCoy, H. Virginia, Kipp, C. William, and Ahern, Melissa (1992). Reducing older patients' reliance on the emergency department. *Social Work in Health Care,* 17(1): 23-37.

Morrow-Howell, Nancy and Proctor, Enola (1994). Discharge destinations of Medicare patients receiving discharge planning: Who goes where? *Medical Care,* 32(5): 486-497.

Nacman, Martin (1977). Social work in health settings: A historical review. *Social Work in Health Care,* 2(4): 407-418.

National Association of Social Workers (1987). NASW standards for social work in health care settings. Washington, DC: NASW Press, 3-30.

National Association of Social Workers (1990). NASW clinical indicators for social work and psychosocial services in the acute care medical hospital. Washington, DC: NASW Press, 1-8.

National Association of Social Workers (1997). Government relations alert: Large volume of letters needed to convince HCFA to retain definition of qualified social workers in Medicare's home health program. Washington, DC: National Association of Social Workers, Web site, March 31.

Oktay, Julianne S., Steinwachs, Donald M., Manon, Joyce, Bone, Lee R., and Fahey, Maureen (1992). Evaluating social work discharge planning services for elderly people: Access, complexity, and outcome. *Health and Social Work,* 17(4): 290-298.

Ortiz, Elizabeth Thompson and Bassoff, Betty Z. (1988). Proprietary hospital social work. *Health and Social Work,* 13(2)(Spring): 114-121.

Ponto, Jade M. and Berg, William (1992). Social work services in the emergency department: A cost-benefit analysis of an extended coverage program. *Health and Social Work,* 17(1): 66-73.

Pray, Jackie E. (1991). Responding to psychosocial needs: Physician perceptions of their referral practices for hospitalized patients. *Health and Social Work,* 16(3): 184-192.

Proctor, Enola K., Morrow-Howell, Nancy, Kitchen, Alice, and Wang, Yeong-Tsyr (1995). Pediatric discharge planning: Complications, efficiency, and adequacy. *Social Work in Health Care,* 22(1): 1-18.

Rauch, Julia B. and Schreiber, Hanita (1985). Discharge planning as a teaching mechanism. *Health and Social Work,* 10(3): 208-216.

Resnick, Cheryl and Dziegielewski, Sophia F. (1996). The relationship between therapeutic termination and job satisfaction among medical social workers. *Social Work in Health Care,* 23(3): 17-32.

Robinson, James C. (1994). The changing boundaries of the American hospital. *The Milbank Quarterly*, 72(2): 259-275. (Quoted material reprinted with permission of Blackwell Publishers, Malden, MA.)

Rosen, George (1958). *A history of public health*. MD monographs on medical history. New York: MD Publications.

Ross, Judith W. (1993). Editorial. Redefining hospital social work: An embattled professional domain. *Health and Social Work*, 18(4): 243-246.

Ross, Judith W. (1995). Hospital social work. In Edwards, Richard L. (Ed.), *The Encyclopedia of Social Work*, (Nineteenth edition). Washington, DC: NASW Press, 1365-1377.

Ruster, Pamela L. (1995). The evolution of social work in a community hospital. *Social Work in Health Care*, 20(4): 73-88.

Showers, Nancy (1992). How satisfaction with hospital field work affects social work student's willingness to accept employment in hospital settings. *Social Work in Health Care*, 16(4): 19-35.

Smith, David R. and Anderson, Ron J. (1995). Feudal vs. futile medicine: Can we have cost containment without prevention? In Eve, Susan Brown, Havens, Betty, and Ingman, Stanley E. (Eds.), *The Canadian health care system: Lessons for the United States*. Lanham, MD: University Press of America, 247-255.

Soskolne, Varda and Auslander, Gail K. (1993). Follow-up evaluation of discharge planning by social workers in an acute-care medical center in Israel. *Social Work in Health Care*, 18(2): 22-48.

Spitzer, William and Burke, Laurie (1993). Practice forum: A critical incident stress debriefing program for hospital-based health care personnel. *Health and Social Work*, 18(2): 149-156.

Spitzer, William and Neely, Keith (1992). Critical incident stress: The role of hospital-based social work in developing a statewide intervention system for first-responders delivering emergency services. *Social Work in Health Care*, 18(1): 39-58.

Stuen, Cynthia and Monk, Abraham (1990). Discharge planning: The impact of Medicare's prospective payment on elderly patients. In A. Monk (Ed.), *Health care of the aged: Needs, policies and services* (pp. 149-164). Binghamton, NY: The Haworth Press.

Task Force on Adolescent Assault Victim Needs (1996). Adolescent assault victim needs: A review of issues and a model protocol. *Pediatrics*, 98(5): 991-1001.

Trattner, Walter I. (1989). *From poor law to welfare state: A history of social welfare in America* (Fourth edition). New York: The Free Press.

Travis, Shirley S., Moore, Suzanne R., and McAuley, William J. (1991). A comparison of hospitalization experiences for demented and nondemented elders: Findings of a retrospective chart review. *Journal of Gerontological Social Work*, 17(1/2): 35-46.

U.S. Government Printing Office (1995a). *Health, United States*. Washington, DC: Author.

U.S. Government Printing Office (1995b). *Statistical Abstracts of the United States, 1995*. Washington, DC: Author.

Walsh, Susan (1985). The psychiatric emergency service as a setting for social work training. *Social Work in Health Care,* 11(1): 21-31.

Wolock, Isabel, Schlesinger, Elfriede, Dinerman, Miriam, and Seaton, Richard (1987). The posthospital needs and care of patients: Implications for discharge planning. *Social Work in Health Care,* 12(4): 6176.

Chapter 5

Applewhite, Steven Lozano (1995). Curanderismo: Demystifying the health beliefs and practices of elderly Mexican-Americans. *Health and Social Work,* 20(4): 247-253.

Aranda, Maria P. (1996). *Implications of diversity for practice.* Presented on June 18, 1996 at the California Geriatric Education Center, Cultural Diversity in Aging, Faculty Development Program, UCLA.

Balinsky, Warren (1994). *Home care.* San Francisco, CA: Jossey-Bass Publishers.

Barnes, Carla L., Given, Barbara A., and Given, Charles W. (1992). Caregivers of elderly relatives: Spouses and adult children. *Health and Social Work,* 17(4): 282-289.

Berkman, Barbara (1996). The emerging health care world: Implications for social work practice and education. *Social Work,* 41(5): 541-555.

Binney, Elizabeth A., Estes, Carroll L., and Ingman, Stanley R. (1990). Medicalization, public policy and the elderly: Social services in jeopardy? *Social Science in Medicine,* 30(7): 761-771.

Blazer, Dan (1988). Home health care: House calls revisited. *American Journal of Public Health,* 78(3): 238-239.

Braus, Patricia (1994). When mom needs help. *American Demographics,* 16 (March): 38-47.

Brody, Elaine M. (1981). Women in the middle and family help to older people. *The Gerontologist,* 21(5): 471-480.

Cannon, Ida M. (1923). *Social work in hospitals.* New York: Russell Sage.

Chadiha, Letha A., Proctor, Enola K., Morrow-Howell, Nancy, Darkwa, Osei K., and Dore, Peter (1995). Post-hospital home care for African-American and white elderly. *The Gerontologist,* 35(2): 233-239.

Clemen-Stone, Susan H., Eigsti, Diane G., and McGuire, Sandra L. (1987). *Comprehensive family and community health nursing* (Second edition). New York: McGraw-Hill.

Corin, Ellen E. (1994). The social and cultural matrix of health and disease. In Evans, Robert G., Barer, Morris L., and Marmor, Theodore R. (Eds.), *Why are some people healthy and others not? The determinants of health of populations.* New York: Aldine de Gruyter, 93-132.

Cox, Carole (1992). Expanding social work's role in home care: An ecological perspective. *Social Work,* 37(2): 179-183.

Damon-Rodriguez, JoAnn, Wallace, Steven, and Kington, Raynard (1994). Service utilization and minority elderly: Appropriateness, accessibility, and acceptability. In Wieland, Daryl, Benton, Donna, Kramer, B. Josea, and Dawson, Grace D.

(Eds.), *Cultural diversity and geriatric care: Challenges to the health profes-sions.* Binghamton, NY: The Haworth Press, Inc., 45-63.

Davitt, Joan K. and Kaye, Lenard W. (1996). Supporting patient autonomy in home health care. *Social Work,* 41(1): 41-50.

Duke University Center for the Study of Aging and Human Development (1978). *The OARS methodology* (Second edition). Durham, NC: Duke University Press.

Ell, Kathleen (1996). Social work and health care practice and policy: A psycho-social research agenda. *Social Work,* 41(6): 583-592.

Erikson, Eric (1950). The problem of ego identity. *Psychological Issues,* 101-164.

Erikson, Eric (1956). The problems of ego identity. *The Journal of the American Psychoanalytic Association,* 4, 56-121.

Erikson, Eric (1959). Identity and the life cycle. In Klein, George S. (Ed.), *Psycho-logical Issues.* Independence, MD: International Universities Press, 56-121.

Ettner, Susan L. (1994). The effect of the Medicaid home care benefit on long-term care choices of the elderly. *Economic Inquiry* (XXXII) January: 103-127.

Fandetti, Donald V. and Goldmeier, John (1988). Social workers as culture media-tors in health care settings. *Health and Social Work,* 13(3) (Summer): 171-179.

Fashimpar, Gary (1983). A management tool for evaluating the adequacy and quality of homemaker-home health aide programs. *The Gerontologist,* 23(2): 127-131.

Fashimpar, Gary (1991). Evaluating homemaker-home health aide programs: Prac-tical applications of the homemaker-home health aide program evaluation ques-tionnaire. *Journal of Gerontological Social Work,* 18(1/2): 3-16.

Fessler, Susan R. and Adams, Catherine G. (1985). Nurse/social worker role con-flict in home health care. *Journal of Gerontological Social Work,* 9(1): 113-123.

Fredman, Lisa, Droge, Janet, and Rabin, David (1992). Functional limitations among home health care users in the national health interview survey supple-ment on aging. *The Gerontologist,* 32(5): 641-646.

Garner, Dianne J. (1995). Long-term care. In Edwards, Richard L. (Ed.), *The Encyclopedia of Social Work* (Nineteenth edition). Washington, DC: NASW Press.

Ginsberg, Leon (1995). *The Social work almanac* (Second edition). Washington, DC: NASW Press.

Giordano, Joseph (1992). Ethnicity and aging. In Mellor, M. Joanna and Solomon, Renee (Eds.), *Geriatric Social Work Education.* Binghamton, NY: The Haworth Press, Inc., 23-37.

Goldberg, Allen J. (1994). Book reviews: Home health care—An annotated bibli-ography. *Journal of the American Geriatric Society,* 42(8): 910-911.

Horowitz, A. (1984). Family caregiving to the frail elderly. In Eisdorfer, Carl (Ed.), *The annual review of gerontology and geriatrics.* New York: Springer, 194-246.

Jacobs, Phillip E. and Lurie, Abraham (1984). A new look at home care and the hospital social worker. In Dobrof, Rose (Ed.), *Gerontological Social Work in Home Health Care.* Binghamton, NY: The Haworth Press, Inc., 89-90.

Jette, Alan M., Smith, Kevin W., and McDermott, Susan M. (1996). Quality of Medicare-reimbursed home health care. *The Gerontologist,* 36(4): 492-501.

Kane, Robert L., Finch, Michael, Blewett, Lynn, Chen, Qing, Burns, Risa, and Moskowitz, Mark (1996). Use of post-hospital care by Medicare patients. *Journal of the American Geriatric Society*, 44(3): 242-250.

Kane, Robert L., Kane, Rosalie A., Finch, Michael, Harrington, Charlene, Newcomer, Robert, Miller, Nancy, and Hulbert, Melissa (1997). S/HMO's, the second generation: Building on the experience of the first social health maintenance organization demonstrations. *Journal of the American Geriatric Society*, 45(1): 101-107.

Karger, Howard Jacob and Stoesz, David. (1994). *American social welfare policy: A pluralistic approach,* (Second edition). New York and London: Longman.

Kaye, Lenard W. and Davitt, Joan K. (1995). Provider and consumer profiles of traditional and high-tech home health care. *Health and Social Work*, 20(4): 262-271.

Kenney, Genevieve M. (1993). Is access to home health care a problem in rural areas? *American Journal of Public Health*, 83(3): 412-414.

Kerson, Toba Schwaber and Michelson, Renee W. (1995). Counseling homebound clients and their families. *Journal of Gerontological Social Work*, 24(3/4): 159-190.

Kramer, Andrew M., Shaughnessy, Peter W., Bauman, Marjorie K., and Crisler, Kathryn S. (1990). Assessing and assuring the quality of home health care: A conceptual framework. *The Milbank Quarterly*, 68(3): 413-443.

Lawlor, Edward F. and Raube, Kristiana (1995). Social interventions and outcomes in medical effectiveness research. *Social Service Review*, 69(3)(September): 383-404. (Quoted material reprinted with permission of University of Chicago Press, Chicago, IL.)

Linsk, Nathan, Keigher, Sharon M., and Osterbusch, Suzanne E. (1988). States' policies regarding paid family caregiving. *The Gerontologist*, 28(2): 204-212.

Mailick, Mildred D., and Jordon, Pearl (1977). A multimodal approach to collaborative practice in acute care hospitals. *Social Work in Health Care*, 2(4): 445-455.

Marder, Reggi and Linsk, Nathan L. (1995). Addressing AIDS long-term care issues through education and advocacy. *Health and Social Work*, 20(1): 75-80.

McCormick, Wayne C., Uomoto, Jay, Young, Heather, Graves, Amy B., Vitaliano, Peter, Mortimer, James. A., Edland, Steven D., and Larson, Eric B. (1996). Attitudes toward use of nursing homes and home care in older Japanese-Americans. *Journal of the American Geriatric Society*, 44(7): 769-777.

Mindel, Charles and Wright, Roosevelt (1982). Satisfaction in multigenerational households. *Journal of Gerontology*, 37(4): 483-489.

Moody, Harry (1982). Ethical dilemmas in long-term care. *Journal of Gerontological Social Work*, 5(1/2): 97-111.

Morrow-Howell, Nancy, Chadiha, Letha A., Proctor, Enola K., Hourd-Bryant, Maggie, and Dore, Peter (1996). Racial differences in discharge planning. *Health and Social Work*, 21(2): 131-139.

National Association for Home Care (1996). *Basic statistics about home care.* Washington, DC: Author.

National Association for Home Care (1997). *Basic statistics about home care.* Washington, DC: NAHC home page: <www.NAHC.org/consumer/hcstats.html>.

National Association of Social Workers (1987). NASW standards for social work in health care settings. Washington DC: NASW Press, 1-31.

National Association of Social Workers (1995). NASW clinical indicators for social work and psychosocial services in home health care. Washington, DC: NASW Press, 1-9.

Olson, Laura Katz (1994). Public policy and privatization: Long-term care in the United States. In Olson, Laura Katz (Ed.), *The graying of the world: Who will care for the frail elderly?* Binghamton, NY: The Haworth Press, Inc., 25-58.

Proctor, Enola K., Morrow-Howell, Nancy, and Kaplan, Sally J. (1996). Implementation of discharge plans for chronically ill elders discharged home. *Health and Social Work*, 21(1): 30-39.

Reamer, Frederic G. and Abramson, Marcia (1982). *The teaching of social work ethics.* Hastings on Hudson, NY: Institute of Society, Ethics, and the Life Sciences.

Robbins, Dennis, A. (1996). *Ethical and legal issues in home health and long-term care: Challenges and solutions.* Gaithersburg, MD: Aspen Publishers.

Silverstone, Barbara and Burack-Weiss, Ann (1982). The social work function in nursing homes and home care. *The Journal of Gerontological Social Work*, 5(1/2): 7-33.

Simmons, June (1994). Community based care: The new health social work paradigm. *Social Work in Health Care*, 20(1): 35-46.

Tanjasiri, Sora P., Wallace, Steven P., and Shibata, Kazue (1995). Picture imperfect: Hidden problems among Asian Pacific Islander elderly. *The Gerontologist*, 35(6): 753-760.

U.S. Department of Health and Human Services, National Institute of Health, National Institute on Aging (1993). *Profiles of America's Elderly: Racial and Ethnic Diversity of America's Elderly Population.* Number 3, November, POP/93-1-8.

U.S. Government Printing Office (1995a). *Health, United States.* Washington, DC: Author.

U.S. Government Printing Office (1995b). *Statistical Abstracts of the United States.* Washington, DC: Author.

Wallace, Steven P. (1990). The political economy of health care for elderly blacks. *International Journal of Health Services*, 20(4): 665-680.

Wallace, Steven P. (1996). *Stratification, ethnicity, and aging public policy.* Presented on June 18, 1996 at the the California Geriatric Education Center, Cultural Diversity in Aging, Faculty Development Program, UCLA.

Ware, John E. and Sherbourne (1992). The MOS 36-item short-form health survey (SF-36). *Medical Care,* 30(6)(June): 473-483.

Welch, H. Gilbert, Wennberg, David E., and Welch, W. Pete (1996). The use of Medicare home health care services. *The New England Journal of Medicine,* 335(5)(August 1): 324-329.

White-Means, Shelly I. and Thornton, Michael C. (1990a). Ethnic differences in the production of informal home health care. *The Gerontologist*, 30(6): 758-768.

White-Means, Shelly I. and Thornton, Michael C. (1990b). Labor market choices and home health care provision among employed ethnic caregivers. *The Gerontologist*, 30(6): 769-775.

Wilcox, Julie A. and Taber, Merlin A. (1991). Informal helpers of elderly home care clients. *Health and Social Work*, 16(4): 258-265.

Zimmer, James G., Groth-Juncker, Annemarie, and McCusker, Jane (1985). A randomized controlled study of a home health care team. *The American Journal of Public Health*, 75(2): 134-141.

Chapter 6

Barber, Clinton E. and Iwai, Mieko (1996). Role conflict and role ambiguity as predictors of burnout among staff caring for elderly dementia patients. *Journal of Gerontological Social Work*, 26(1/2): 101-117.

Beirne, Nancy F., Patterson, Margery N., Galie, Michelle, and Goodman, Patricia (1995). Effects of a fast-tract closing on a nursing facility population. *Health and Social Work*, 20(2): 117-123.

Bogo, Marion (1987). Social work practice with family systems in admission to homes for the aged. *Journal of Gerontological Social Work*, 10(1/2): 5-19.

Boondas, Jennifer (1991). Nursing home resident assessment classification and focused care. *Nursing and Health Care*, 12(6): 308-312.

Brannon, Diane (1992). Toward second-generation nursing home research. *The Gerontologist*, 32(3): 293-294. (Quoted material reprinted with permission of The Gerontological Society of America, Washington, DC.)

Brown, Lil (1989). Is there sexual freedom for our aging population in long-term care institutions? *Journal of Gerontological Social Work*, 13(3/4): 75-93.

Bruno, Ronald (1994). Policy for the people: One facility's introduction to restraint reduction. *Journal of Gerontological Social Work*, 22(3/4): 129-142.

Bullard-Poe, Laura, Powell, Cicely, and Mulligan, Thomas (1994). The importance of intimacy to men living in a nursing home. *Archives of Sexual Behavior*, 23(2): 231-236.

Caplan, Arthur L. (1990). The morality of the mundane: Ethical issues arising in the daily lives of nursing home residents. In Kane, Rosalie A. and Caplan, Arthur L. (Eds.), *Everyday ethics: Resolving dilemmas in nursing home life*. New York: Springer, 37-50.

Cohen-Mansfield, Jiska, Rabinovich, Beth A., Marx, Marcia S., Braun, Judith, and Fleshner, Edith (1991). Nurses' and social workers' perceptions of elderly nursing home residents' well-being. *Journal of Gerontological Social Work*, 16(3/4): 135-147.

Cox, Carole (1993). Dealing with the aggressive nursing home resident. *Journal of Gerontological Social Work*, 19(3/4): 179-192.

Dane, B.O. and Simon, B.L. (1991). Resident guests: Social workers in host settings. *Social Work*, 36: 208-213.

Dempsey, Norah P. and Pruchno, Rachel A. (1993). The family's role in the nursing home: Predictors of technical and non-technical assistance. *Journal of Gerontological Social Work*, 21(1/2): 127-145.

Dhooper, Surjit S., Green, Sharon M., Huff, Marlene B., and Austin-Murphy, Judy (1993). Efficacy of a group approach to reducing depression in nursing home residents. *Journal of Gerontological Social Work*, 20(3/4): 87-100.

Dieckmann, Janna L. (1993). From almshouse to city nursing home: Philadelphia's Riverview home for the aged, 1945-1965. *Nursing History Review*, 1: 217-228.

Evans, L. and Strump, F. (1989). Tying down the elderly: A review of the literature on physical restraint. *Journal of the American Geriatrics Society*, 37(1): 65-74.

Fairchild, Susan, Carrino, Gerard E., and Ramirez, Mildred (1996). Social workers' perceptions of staff attitudes toward resident sexuality in a random sample of New York State nursing homes. *Journal of Gerontological Social Work*, 26(1/2): 153-169.

Foldes, Steven S. (1990). Life in an institution: A sociological and anthropological view. In Kane, Rosalie A. and Caplan, Arthur L. (Eds.), *Everyday ethics: Resolving dilemmas in nursing home life*. New York: Springer, 21-36.

Freed, Anne O. (1990) How Japanese families cope with fragile elderly. *Journal of Gerontological Social Work*, 15(1/2): 39-56.

Freeman, Iris C. (1988). "Weighing the costs of care," in Point/Counterpoint: Caring for persons with aids in geriatric nursing homes. *Health and Social Work*, 13(2)(Spring), 156-158.

Getzel, Jessica (1983). Resident councils and social action. In Getzel, George S. and Mellor, M. Joanna (Eds.), *Gerontological social work practice in long-term care*. Binghamton, NY: The Haworth Press, Inc., 179-185.

Greene, Roberta, Vourlekis, Betsy S., Gelfand, Donald, and Lewis, Judith S. (1992). Current realities: Practice and education needs of social workers in nursing homes. *Journal of Gerontological Social Work*, 18(3/4): 39-54.

Gutheil, Irene (1991). Intimacy in nursing home friendships. *Journal of Gerontological Social Work*, 17(1/2): 59-73.

Hancock, Tina U. (1992). Field placements in for-profit organizations: Policies and practices of graduate programs. *Journal of Social Work Education*, 28(3): 330-340.

Health Care Financing Administration (1989). *Medicare and Medicaid data book 1988*. HCFA publication number 03270. Baltimore, MD: Office of Research and Demonstrations.

Hoffman, Rosemary G. (1991). Companion animals: A therapeutic measure for elderly patients. *Journal of Gerontological Social Work*, 18(1/2): 195-204.

Horejsi, Gloria (1987). Nursing home consultation. *Health and Social Work*, Spring, 12(2): 155-156.

Institute of Medicine (1981). *Health care in a context of civil rights*. Washington, DC: National Academy Press.

Joint Commission on the Accreditation of Healthcare Organizations (1993). *Accreditation Manual for Long Term Care: 1994, Volume 1, Organization Standards*. Oak Brook Terrace, IL: JCAHO.

Kaas, M.J. (1978). Sexual expression of the elderly in nursing homes. *The Gerontologist*, 18(4): 372-378.

Kane, Rosalie A. and Caplan, Arthur L. (Eds.) (1990). *Everyday ethics: Resolving dilemmas in nursing home life.* New York: Springer.

Karger, Howard Jacob and Stoesz, David (1994). *American social welfare policy: A pluralistic approach* (Second edition). New York: Longman.

Kruzich, Jean M. (1995). Empowering organizational contexts: Patterns and predictors of perceived decision-making influence among staff in nursing homes. *The Gerontologist*, 35(2): 207-216.

Kruzich, Jean M. and Powell, William E. (1995). Decision-making influence: An empirical study of social workers in nursing homes. *Health and Social Work*, 20(3): 215-222.

Lerer, Gertie (1995). Helping the irascible patient in long term care: Toward a theoretical and practice design. *Journal of Gerontological Social Work*, 24(1/2): 169-184.

Linsk, Nathan L. and Marder, Reggi E. (1992). Medical social work long term care referrals for people with HIV infection. *Health and Social Work*, 17(2): 105-115.

Margolis, Richard J. (1990). *Risking old age in America.* Westview Press, Boulder, Colorado.

Mead, Nelson B. (1991). Some nursing home experiences. *Journal of Gerontological Social Work*, 16(3/4): 3-15.

Mercer, Susan O. (1996). Navaho elderly people in a reservation nursing home: Admission predictors and culture care practices. *Social Work*, 41(2): 181-189.

Mercer, Susan O. (1994). Navajo elders in a reservation nursing home: Health status profile. *Journal of Gerontological Social Work*, 23(1/2): 3-29.

Monahan, Deborah J. (1995). Informal caregivers of institutionalized demential residents: Predictors of burden. *Journal of Gerontological Social Work*, 23(3/4): 65-82.

Montgomery, Rhonda J.V. and Kosloski, Karl (1994). A longitudinal analysis of nursing home placement for dependent elders care for by spouses vs. adult children. *Journal of Gerontology*, 49(2): S62-S74.

Morrison, Barbara Jones (1995). A research and policy agenda on predictors of institutional placement among minority elderly. *Journal of Gerontological Social Work*, 24(1/2): 17-28.

Morrow-Howell, Nancy, Chadiha, Letha A., Proctor, Enola K., Hourd-Bryant, Maggie, and Dore, Peter (1996). Racial differences in discharge planning. *Health and Social Work*, 21(2): 131-139.

Mosher-Ashley, Pearl M., Turner, Barbara F., and O'Neill, Darcy (1991). Attitudes of nursing and rest home administrators toward deinstitutionalized elders with psychiatric disorders. *Community Mental Health Journal*, 27(4): 241-253.

National Association of Social Workers (1981). NASW standards for social work services in long-term care facilities. Washington, DC: NASW Press, 1-11.

National Association of Social Workers (1993). NASW clinical indicators for social work and psychosocial services in nursing homes. Washington, DC: NASW Press, 1-12.

Nelson, Wayne H. (1995). Long-term care volunteer roles on trial: Ombudsman effectiveness revisited. *Journal of Gerontological Social Work*, 23(3/4): 25-46.

Olson, Laura Katz (1994). Public policy and privatization: Long-term care in the United States. In Olson, Laura Katz (Ed.), *The graying of the world: Who will care for the frail elderly?* Binghamton, NY: The Haworth Press, Inc., 25-58.

Palmer, Diane S. (1991). Co-leading a family council in a long-term care facility. *Journal of Gerontological Social Work*, 16(3/4): 121-134.

Pepper Commission. U.S. Bipartisan Commission on Comprehensive Health Care (1990). *A call for action: Final report.* Washington, DC: U.S. Government Printing Office.

Quam, Jean K. and Whitford, Gary S. (1992). Educational needs of nursing home social workers at the baccalaureate level. *Journal of Gerontological Social Work*, 18(3/4): 143-156.

Reinardy, James R. (1995). Relocation to a new environment: Decisional control and the move to a nursing home. *Health and Social Work*, 20(1): 31-38.

Riddick, Carol Cutler, Cohen-Mansfield, Jiska, Fleshner, Edith, and Kraft, Gladys (1992). Caregiver adaptations to having a relative with dementia admitted to a nursing home. *Journal of Gerontological Social Work*, 19(1): 51-75.

Salive, Marcel E., Collins, Karen S., Foley, Daniel J., and George, Linda K. (1993). Predictors of nursing home admission in a biracial population. *American Journal of Public Health*, 83(12): 1765-1767.

Scharlach, Andrew (1988). Peer counselor training for nursing home residents. *The Gerontologist*, 28(4): 500-502.

Silverstone, Barbara and Burack-Weiss, Ann (1982). The social work function in nursing homes and home care. *The Journal of Gerontological Social Work*, 5(1/2): 7-33.

Smith, David Barton (1990). Population ecology and the racial integration of hospitals and nursing homes in the United States. *The Milbank Quarterly*, 68(4): 561-596.

Spears, Renee, Drinka, Paul J., and Voeks, Susan K. (1993). Obtaining a durable power of attorney for health care from nursing home residents. *The Journal of Family Practice*, 36(4): 409-413.

Tennstedt, Sharon L., Skinner, Katherine M., Sullivan, Lisa M., and McKinlay, John B. (1992). Response comparability of family and staff proxies for nursing home residents. *American Journal of Public Health*, 82(5): 747-749.

U.S. Civil Rights Commission (1963). *Civil rights: Report of the United States Civil Rights Commission.* Washington, DC: U.S. Government Printing Office.

U.S. Government Printing Office (1990). *Developments in Aging: 1990* (Volume 1). Washington, DC: U.S. Senate Special Committee on Aging.

U.S. Government Printing Office (1994/1995). *Social Security Bulletin, Annual Statistical Supplement, 1994 and 1995.* Washington, DC: Author.

U.S. Government Printing Office (1995a). *Health United States,* Washington, DC: Author.

U.S. Government Printing Office (1995b). *Statistical Abstracts of the United States.* Washington, DC: Author.

Vinton, Linda and Mazza, Nicholas (1994). Aggressive behavior directed at nursing home personnel by residents' family members. *The Gerontologist*, 34(4): 528-533.

Vogel, William (1991). A personal memoir of the state hospitals of the 1950's. *Hospital and Community Psychiatry*, 42(6): 593-597.

Vourlekis, Betsy S., Gelfand, Donald E., and Greene, Roberta R. (1992). Psychosocial needs and care in nursing homes: Comparison of views of social workers and home administrators. *The Gerontologist*, 32(1): 113-119. (Copyright © The Gerontological Society of America. Reproduced by permission of the publisher.)

Wards Business Directory of U.S. Private and Public Companies (1997) (Volume 5). Detroit, MI: Gale Publishing Company.

Wasow, Mona and Loeb, Martin (1979). Sexuality in nursing homes. *Journal of the American Geriatrics Society*, 27, 73-79.

Weisberg, Judith (1991). Social worker as client: My education as a family member in a nursing home. *Journal of Gerontological Social Work*, 16(1/2): 195-203.

Williams, Ann (1997). American Healthcare Association spokesperson. Phone conversation with author, July 23, 1997.

Williams, Carter C. (1989). Liberation: Alternative to physical restraints. *The Gerontologist*, 29(5): 385-386.

Wullschleger, Karla Scroggin, Lund, Dale A., Caserta, Michael S., and Wright, Scott D. (1996). Anxiety about aging: A neglected dimension of caregivers' experience. *Journal of Gerontological Social Work*, 26(3/4): 3-18.

Chapter 7

Allison, Helen, Gripton, James, and Rodway, Margaret (1990). Social work services as a component of palliative care with terminal cancer patients. In Davidson, Kay W. and Clarke, Sylvia S. (Eds.), *Social work in health care: A handbook for practice. Part I*. Binghamton, NY: The Haworth Press, Inc., 205-223.

Amar, Deborah F. (1994). The role of the hospice social worker in the nursing home setting. *The American Journal of Hospice and Palliative Care*, 11(3)(May/June): 18-22.

Buckingham, Robert W. (1996). *The handbook of hospice care*. New York: Prometheus Books.

Cassell, Eric (1982). The nature of suffering and the goals of medicine. *The New England Journal of Medicine*, 306: 639-645.

Corbett, Terry L. and Hai, Dorothy M. (1979). Searching for euthanatos: The hospice alternative. *Hospital Progress*, 60(3): 38-41.

Corr, Charles and Corr, Donna (1985). Situations involving children: A challenge for the hospice movement. *The Hospice Journal*, 1(2): 63-77.

Donovan, Jenny A. (1984). Team nurse and social worker: Avoiding role conflict. *American Journal of Hospice Care*, 1(1): 21-23.

Doyle, Derek (1994). Domiciliary palliative care: A guide for the primary care team. Oxford, New York, Tokyo: Oxford University Press.

Dush, David M. (1988a). Psychosocial research in hospice care: Toward a specificity of therapeutic mechanisms. *The Hospice Journal*, 4(2): 9-36.

Dush, David M. (1988b). Trends in hospice research and psychosocial palliative care. *The Hospice Journal*, 4(3): 13-28.

Fish, Nina Millet (1994). Social work practice in hospice care. In Holosko, M.J. and Taylor, P.A. (Eds.), *Social work practice in health care settings*. Toronto, Canada: Canadian Scholar's Press, 403-418.

Freund, Peter E.S. and McGuire, Meridith B. (1991). *Health, illness and the social body: A critical sociology*. Englewood Cliffs, NJ: Prentice-Hall.

Germain, Carel Bailey (1984). *Social work practice in health care: An ecological perspective*. New York: The Free Press.

Gummer, Burton (1988). The hospice in transition: organizational and administrative perspectives. In F.D. Perlmutter (Ed.), *Alternative social agencies: Administrative strategies*. Binghamton, NY: The Haworth Press, 31-43.

Hayslip, Bert and Leon, Joel (1992). *Hospice care*. Newbury Park, CA: Sage Publications.

Kaye, Lenard W. and Davitt, Joan K. (1995). Provider and consumer profiles of traditional and high-tech home health care. *Health and Social Work*, 20(4): 262-271.

Kerr, Derek, M.D. (1993). Mother Mary Aikenhead, the Irish Sisters of Charity and Our Lady's Hospice for the Dying. *The American Journal of Hospice and Palliative Care*, 10(3)(May/June): 13-20.

Kron, Joan (1978). Designing a better place to die. In Swartz, Howard D. and Kart, Cary S. (Eds.), *Dominant issues in medical sociology*. Reading, MA: Addison-Wesley, 548-554.

Kübler-Ross, Elisabeth (1969). *On death and dying*. New York: Macmillan.

Kulys, R. and Davis, M. (1986). An analysis of social services in hospice. *Social Work*, 31(6): 448-456.

Lusk, Mark (1983). The psychosocial evaluation of the hospice patient. *Health and Social Work*, 8(3): 210-218.

McDonald, Douglas (1991). Hospice social work: A search for identity. *Health and Social Work*, 16(4): 274-280.

McNulty, Elizabeth G. and Holderby, Robert A. (1983). *Hospice: A caring challenge*. Springfield, IL: Charles C Thomas.

Moore, Kathleen (1984). Training social workers to work with the terminally ill. *Health and Social Work*, 19(4): 268-273.

Mount, Balfour (1993). Whole person care: Beyond psychosocial and physical needs. *The American Journal of Hospice and Palliative Care*, (January/February): 28-37.

National Association for Home Care (1996). *Basic statistics about home care*, Washington, DC: Author, 11 pp.

Paradis, Lenora Finn (1985). *Hospice handbook: A guide for managers and planners*. Rockford, MD: Aspen Systems.

Parry, Joan K. and Ryan, Angela Shen (Eds.) (1995). *A cross-cultural look at death, dying, and religion*. Chicago, IL: Nelson Hall.

Phipps, E.E. (1988). The origin of hospices/hospitals. *Death Studies*, 12(2): 91-99.

Pilsecker, C. (1979). Terminal cancer: A challenge for social work. *Social Work in Health Care*, 4(4): 369-379.

Preston, Robert (1979). *The dilemmas of care.* New York: Elsevier Press.

Proffitt, Linda J. (1987). Hospice. In Minahan, Anne (Ed.), *The Encyclopedia of Social Work* (Eighteenth edition). Washington, DC: NASW Press, 812-816.

Quig, L. (1989). The role of the hospice social worker. *American Journal of Hospice Care*, 6(4): 22-23.

Rodway, Margaret R. and Blythe, Judith (1994). Social work practice in palliative care. In Holosko, M.J. and Taylor, P.A. (Eds.), *Social Work Practice in Health Care Settings.* Toronto, Canada: Canadian Scholar's Press, 419-437.

Richman, Jack M. (1995). Hospice. In Edwards, Richard L. (Ed.), *The Encyclopedia of Social Work* (Nineteenth edition). Washington, DC: NASW Press, 1358-1364.

Rusnack, Betty, Schaefer, Sarajane McNulty, and Moxley, David (1988). "Safe passage": Social work roles and functions in hospice care. *Social Work in Health Care*, 13(3): 3-18.

Saunders, Cicely (1982). Hospice care. In Ajemian, Ina and Mount, Balfour (Eds.), *The R.V.H. manual on pallative hospice care: A resource manual.* Salem, NH: Ayer, 21-26.

Smith, Wade (1994). Building a hospice: A personal viewpoint. In Kornblum, William and Smith, Carolyn D. (Eds.), *The healing experience: Readings on the social context of health care.* Englewood Cliffs, NY: Prentice-Hall, 203-208.

Sontag, Mary-Ann (1996). A comparison of hospice programs based on Medicare certification status. *The American Journal of Hospice and Palliative Care*, 13(2) (March/April): 32-41.

Sontag, Mary-Ann, Nadig, Jennifer, and Henry, Lisa (1994). The children's grief workshop: Social work practice in hospice. *The American Journal of Hospice and Palliative Care,* 11(3)(May/June): 23-29.

Stark, Doretta E. and Johnson, Edith M. (1983). Implications of hospice concepts for social work practice with oncology patients and their families in an acute care teaching hospital. *Social Work in Health Care*, 9(1): 63-70.

Storey, Porter (1993). Hospice settings around the world. *The American Journal of Hospice and Palliative Care*, 10(4)(July/August): 4-5.

Strang, P. (1992). Emotional and social aspects of cancer pain. *Acta Oncologica*, 31(3): 323-326.

Stubblefield, Kristine S. (1990). A preventive program for bereaved families. In Davidson, Kay W. and Clarke, Sylvia S. (Eds.), *Social work in health care: A handbook for practice. Part I.* Binghamton, NY: The Haworth Press, Inc., 385-400.

U.S. Government Printing Office (1994). State operations manual: Provider certification. Health Care Financing Administration. Transmittal number 265. (Interpretative Guidelines-Hospice; regulation 418.68, tag number 265).

U.S. Government Printing Office (1995). *Statistical abstracts of the United States.* Washington, DC: Author.

Weiner, Herbert (1984). An integrative model of health, illness, and disease. *Health and Social Work*, 9(4): 253-260.

Weisman, Avery D. (1972). *On death and dying—A psychiatric study of the terminally ill.* New York: Behavioral Publications.

Chapter 8

Ball, Robert M. (1996). Medicare's roots: What Medicare's architects had in mind. *Generations*, 20(2)(Summer): 13-19.

Belcher, John R. (1993). The trade-offs of developing a case management model for chronically mentally ill people. *Health and Social Work*, 18(1): 20-31.

Billings, John (1999). Access to health care services. In Kovner, Anthony R. and Jonas, Steven (Eds.), *Health care delivery in the United States.* New York: Springer, 401-438.

Chambliss, Catherine, Pinto, Debra, and McGuigan, Joan (1997). Reactions to managed care among psychologists and social workers. *Psychological Reports*, 80(1): 147-154.

Cornelius, Donald S. (1994). Managed care and social work: Constructing a context and a response. *Social Work in Health Care*, 20(1): 47-63.

Davidson, Jeanette R. and Davidson, Tim (1996). Confidentiality and managed care: Ethical and legal concerns. *Health and Social Work*, 21(3): 208-215.

Freeman, Michael A. and Trabin, Tom (1994). *Managed behavioral health care: History, models, key issues, and future course.* Rockville, MD: U.S. Center for Mental Health Services.

Friedland, Robert B. (1996). Managed care and all of us: The role of managed care in the future. *Generations,* Summer, 20(2): 37-41.

Friedman, Emily (1996). Capitation, integration, and managed care. *Journal of the American Medical Association*, 275(12): 957-962.

Grayson, Mary (1998). An interview with Dick Davidson. *Hospitals and Health Networks,* 73(July 5): 12-16.

Hodge, Melville H. (1996). Health care and America's rolling depression. *Health Care Management Review,* 21(3): 7-12.

Kane, Robert L. (1995). Canadian lessons in health care reform: Reading between the lines. In Eve, Susan Brown, Havens, Betty, and Ingman, Stanley R. (Eds.), *The Canadian health care system: Lessons for the United States.* Lanham, MD: University Press.

Karger, Howard Jacob and Stoesz, Howard (1998). *American social welfare policy: A pluralistic approach* (Third edition). New York: Longman.

Kirkman-Liff, Bradford L. (1996). Health care reform in the Netherlands, Israel, Germany, England, and Sweden. *Generations,* 20(2)(Summer): 65-69.

Kovner, Anthony R. (1999). Health maintenance organizations and managed care. In Kovner, Anthony R. and Jonas, Steven (Eds.), *Health care delivery in the United States,* New York: Springer, 279-302.

Lave, Judith R. (1996). Rethinking Medicare. *Generations,* 20(2) (Summer): 19-23.

Lyons, Barbara, Rowland, Diane, and Hanson, Kristina (1996). Another look at Medicaid. *Generations,* 20(2)(Summer): 24-29.

Manderscheid, Rondals W. and Henderson, Marilyn J. (1998). Federal and state legislative program directions for managed care. In Mullen, Edward J. and Magnabosco, Jennifer L. (Eds.), *Outcomes measurement in the human services: Cross cutting issues and methods.* Washington, DC: NASW Press, 113-123.

Mechanic, David (1999). *Mental health and social policy: The emergence of managed care* (Fourth edition). Boston: Allyn and Bacon.

Mizrahi, Terry (1993). Managed care and managed competition: A primer for social work. *Health and Social Work,* 18(2): 86-91.

Moore, C.W. (1986). *The mediation process: Practical strategies for resolving conflict.* San Francisco: Jossey-Bass.

Munson, Carlton E. (1997). The future of clinical social work and managed cost organizations. *Psychiatric Services,* 48(4): 479-482.

Newhouse, Joseph P. (1996). An iconoclastic view of health care cost containment. *Generations,* 20(2)(Summer): 61-63.

Rachlis, Michael M. (1997). The Canadian experience with public health insurance. In Eve, Susan Brown, Havens, Betty, and Ingman, Stanley R. (Eds.), *The Canadian health care system: Lessons for the United States.* Lanham, MD: University Press, 143-154.

Rovner, Julie (1998). Brace yourself: Expect an explosion of data about medicare's new options. *AARP Bulletin,* September, 39(8): 2, 18.

Schuster, James M., Kern, Edward E., Kane, Vince, Nettleman, Leslie (1994). Changing roles of mental health clinicians in multidisciplinary teams. *Hospital and Community Psychiatry,* 45(12): 1187-1189.

Simmons, Henry E. (1996). The nation's least understood health care problem—The quality of medical care. *Generations,* 20(2)(Summer): 57-61.

Strom-Gottfried, Kimberly (1998a). Informed consent meets managed care. *Health and Social Work,* 23(1): 25-33.

Strom-Gottfried, Kimberly (1998b). Applying a conflict resolution framework to disputes in managed care. *Social Work,* 43(5): 393-401.

U.S. Government Printing Office (1995). *Statistical abstracts of the United States.* Washington, DC: Author.

U.S. Government Printing Office (1997a). *Health, United States, 1996-1997.* Washington, DC: Author.

U.S. Government Printing Office (1997b). *Statistical abstracts of the United States.* Washington, DC: Author.

Woolhandler, Steffie and Himmelstein, David U. (1997). Costs of care and administration at for-profit and other hospitals in the United States. *New England Journal of Medicine,* 336(11): 769-799.

Zis, Michael, Jacobs, Lawrence R., and Shapiro, Robert Y. (1996). The elusive common ground: The politics of public opinion and health care reform. *Generations,* 20(2)(Summer): 7-11.

Chapter 9

Berkman, Barbara (1998). Outcomes measurement for social work research and practice in health care. In Mullen, Edward J. and Magnabosco, Jennifer L.

(Eds.), *Outcomes measurement in the human services: Cross cutting issues and methods.* Washington, DC: NASW Press, 218-223.

Browne, Colette V., Smith, Margaret, Ewalt, Patricia L., and Walker, Duane D. (1996). Advancing social work practice in health care settings: A collaborative partnership for continuing education. *Health and Social Work,* 21(4): 267-276.

Davidson, Kay (1998). Educating students for social work in health care today. In Schamess, Gerald and Lightburn, Anita (Eds.), *Humane managed care.* Washington, DC: NASW Press, 425-429.

Davis, King (1998). Managed health care: Forcing social work to make choices and changes. In Schamess, Gerald and Lightburn, Anita (Eds.), *Humane managed care.* Washington, DC: NASW Press, 409-424.

Ell, Kathleen (1996). Social work and health care practice and policy: A psychosocial research agenda. *Social Work,* 41(6): 583-592.

Keigher, Sharon M. (1997). What role for social work in the new health care practice paradigm? *Health and Social Work,* 22(2): 149-155.

Kelner, M. (1985). Community support networks: Current issues. *Canadian Journal of Public Health,* 76(supplement 1): 69-70.

McDowell, Ian and Newell, Claire (1987). *Measuring health: A guide to rating scales and questionnaires.* New York: Oxford University Press.

Mechanic, David (1978). *Medical sociology.* New York: The Free Press.

Monkman, Marjorie McQueen (1991). Outcome objectives in social work practice: Persons and environment. *Social Work,* 36(3): 253-258.

Munson, Carlton E. (1998). Evolution and trends in the relationship between clinical social work practice and managed cost organizations. In Schamess, Gerald and Lightburn, Anita (Eds.), *Humane managed care.* Washington, DC: NASW Press, 308-324.

Rosenberg, Gary (1998). Social work in a health and mental health managed care environment. In Schamess, Gerald and Lightburn, Anita (Eds.), *Humane managed care* Washington, DC: NASW Press, 3-22.

Spitzer, William J. and Nash, Kermit B. (1996). Educational preparation for contemporary health care social work practice. *Social Work in Health Care,* 24(1/2): 9-34.

Vaghy, Andrea (1998). Report identifies health care issues affecting social work education. *Social Work Education Reporter,* 46(3): 8, 36.

Van Hook, Mary P., Berkman, Barbara, and Dunkle, Ruth (1996). Assessment tools for general health settings: PRIME MD, OARS, and SF-36. *Health and Social Work,* 21(3): 230-234.

Veeder, Nancy W. and Peebles-Wilkins, Wilma (1998). Research needs in managed behavioral health care. In Schamess, Gerald and Lightburn, Anita (Eds.), *Humane managed care.* Washington, DC: NASW Press, 483-504.

Volland, Patricia J. (1996). Social work practice in health care: Looking to the future with a different lens. *Social Work in Health Care,* 24(1/2): 35-51.

Index

Page numbers followed by the letter "t" indicate tables.

SOCIAL WORK APPROACHES TO CONFLICT RESOLUTION: MAKING FIGHTING OBSOLETE by Benyamin Chetkow-Yanoov. (1996). "Presents an examination of the nature and cause of conflict and suggests techniques for coping with conflict." *Journal of Criminal Justice*

FEMINIST THEORIES AND SOCIAL WORK: APPROACHES AND APPLICATIONS by Christine Flynn Salunier. (1996). " An essential reference to be read repeatedly by all educators and practitioners who are eager to learn more about feminist theory and practice: *Nancy R. Hooyman, PhD, Dean and Professor, School of Social Work, University of Washington, Seattle*

THE RELATIONAL SYSTEMS MODEL FOR FAMILY THERAPY: LIVING IN THE FOUR REALITIES by Donald R. Bardill. (1996). "Engages the reader in quiet, thoughtful conversation on the timeless issue of helping families and individuals." *Christian Counseling Resource Review*

SOCIAL WORK INTERVENTION IN AN ECONOMIC CRISIS: THE RIVER COMMUNITIES PROJECT by Martha Baum and Pamela Twiss. (1996). "Sets a standard for universities in terms of the types of meaningful roles they can play in supporting and sustaining communities." *Kenneth J. Jaros, PhD, Director, Public Health Social Work Training Program, University of Pittsburgh*

FUNDAMENTALS OF COGNITIVE-BEHAVIOR THERAPY: FROM BOTH SIDES OF THE DESK by Bill Borcherdt. (1996). "Both beginning and experienced practitioners . . . will find a considerable number of valuable suggestions in Borcherdt's book." *Albert Ellis, PhD, President, Institute for Rational-Emotive Therapy, New York City*

BASIC SOCIAL POLICY AND PLANNING: STRATEGIES AND PRACTICE METHODS by Hobart A. Burch. (1996). "Burch's familiarity with his topic is evident and his book is an easy introduction to the field." *Readings*

THE CROSS-CULTURAL PRACTICE OF CLINICAL CASE MANAGEMENT IN MENTAL HEALTH edited by Peter Manoleas. (1996). "Makes a contribution by bringing together the cross-cultural and clinical case management perspectives in working with those who have serious mental illness." *Disability Studies Quarterly*

FAMILY BEYOND FAMILY: THE SURROGATE PARENT IN SCHOOLS AND OTHER COMMUNITY AGENCIES by Sanford Weinstein. (1995). "Highly recommended to anyone concerned about the welfare of our children and the breakdown of the American family." *Jerold S. Greenberg, EdD, Director of Community Service, College of Health & Human Performance, University of Maryland*

PEOPLE WITH HIV AND THOSE WHO HELP THEM: CHALLENGES, INTEGRATION, INTERVENTION by R. Dennis Shelby. (1995). "A useful and compassionate contribution to the HIV psychotherapy literature." *Public Health*

THE BLACK ELDERLY: SATISFACTION AND QUALITY OF LATER LIFE by Marguerite Coke and James A. Twaite. (1995). "Presents a model for predicting life satisfaction in this population." *Abstracts in Social Gerontology*

BUILDING ON WOMEN'S STRENGTHS: A SOCIAL WORK AGENDA FOR THE TWENTY-FIRST CENTURY edited by Liane V. Davis. (1994). "The most lucid and accessible overview of the related epistemological debates int he social work literature." *Journal of the National Association of Social Workers*

NOW DARE EVERYTHING: TALES OF HIV-RELATED PSYCHOTHERAPY by Steven F. Dansky. (1994). "A highly recommended book for anyone working with persons who are HIV positive. . . . Every library should have a copy of this book." *AIDS Book Review Journal*

INTERVENTION RESEARCH: DESIGN AND DEVELOPMENT FOR HUMAN SERVICE edited by Jack Rothman and Edwin J. Thomas. (1994). "Provides a useful framework for the further examination of methodology for each separate step of such research." *Academic Library Book Review*

CLINICAL SOCIAL WORK SUPERVISION, SECOND EDITION by Carlton E. Munson. (1993). "A useful, thorough, and articulate reference for supervisors and for 'supervisees' who are wanting to understand their supervisor or are looking for effective supervision." *Transactional Analysis Journal*

ELEMENTS OF THE HELPING PROCESS: A GUIDE FOR CLINICIANS by Raymond Fox. (1993). "Filled with helpful hints, creative interventions, and practical guidelines." *Journal of Family Psychotherapy*

IF A PARTNER HAS AIDS: GUIDE TO CLINICAL INTERVENTION FOR RELATIONSHIPS IN CRISIS by R. Dennis Shelby. (1993). " A welcome addition to existing publications about couples coping with AIDS, it offers intervention ideas and strategies to clinicians." *Contemporary Psychology*

GERONTOLOGICAL SOCIAL WORK SUPERVISION by Ann Burack-Weiss and Frances Coyle Brennan. (1991). "The creative ideas in this book will aid supervisors working with students and experienced social workers." *Senior News*

SOCIAL WORK THEORY AND PRACTICE WITH THE TERMINALLY ILL by Joan K. Parry. (1989). "Should be read by all professionals engaged in the provision of health services in hospitals, emergency rooms, and hospices." *Hector B. Garcia, PhD, Professor, San Jose State University School of Social Work*

THE CREATIVE PRACTITIONER: THEORY AND METHODS FOR THE HELPING SERVICES by Bernard Gelfand. (1988). "[Should] be widely adopted by those in the helping services. It could lead to significant positive advances by countless individuals." *Sidney J. Parnes, Trustee Chairperson for Strategic Program Development, Creative Education Foundation, Buffalo, NY*

MANAGEMENT AND INFORMATION SYSTEMS IN HUMAN SERVICES: IMPLICATIONS FOR THE DISTRIBUTION OF AUTHORITY AND DECISION MAKING by Richard K. Caputo. (1987). "A contribution to social work scholarship in that it provides conceptual frameworks that can be used in the design of management information systems." *Social Work*